46 $ 18-

Auricular-Point-Pressing Therapy

Written by	Shan Qiuhua
Translated by	Lu Mingxia
	Xiao Fei

Shandong Science and Technology Press

First Edition 1996
ISBN 7－5331－1833－2

Auricular-Point-Pressing Therapy

Written by Shan Qiuhua
Translated by Lu Mingxia
Xiao Fei
Editor in charge Li Yu

Published by Shandong Science and Technology Press
16 Yuhan Road, Jinan, China 250002
Printed by Shandong Lai Wu Printing House
Distributde by China International Book Trading Corporation
35 Chegongzhuang xilu, Beijing 100044, China
P. O. Box 399, Beijing, China
Prined in the People's Republic of China

Preface

This is one volume of *The Series of Traditional Chinese Medicine for Foreign Readers.*

Auricular-point-pressing therapy is an important component of Traditional Chinese Medicine (TCM). Over several thousand years' medical practice and life experience, Chinese medical workers have accumulated a considerable experience on auricular therapy and have made great contributions to the treatment and prevention of various diseases involving the internal diseases, surgical diseases, gynecological diseases and pediatric diseases. Up to now, in addition to needling with filiform needles, many other methods for stimulating auricular points have developed, such as needle-embedding, electrostimulation, drug injection, auricular moxibustion, laser radiation and point-pressing. Point-pressing is the most widely applied method because of its convenient manipulation, little injury, painlessness, reliable therapeutic effects and easy acceptance by patients. To promote its application, we compile this book on the basis of collection of all the relevant and available data and the author's twenty years experience. We hope it can make a contribution to the health service of all nations over the world.

This book consists of five parts: *Introduction*, *Anatomy of the Auricle*, *Auricular Points*, *Clinical Application of Auricular-point-pressing Therapy*, and *Treatment of Common Diseases.* In the part of *Introduction*, mechanism and characteristics of auricular-point-pressing are introduced; In the part of *Anatomy of the Auricle*, anatomical knowledge of the auricle is explained in detail; In the part of *Auricular Points*, ninety auricular points adopted by

World Health Organization (WHO) and All-China Association of Acupuncture and Moxibustion and some empirical points are introduced concerning the location, function and indication. In the part of *Clinical Application of Auricular-point-pressing Therapy*, principles for point prescription, detecting methods and different pressing approaches are described; and in the part of *Treatment* of *Common Diseases*, nearly eighty diseases are discussed in aspects of clinical manifestations, point selection, pressing methods, basis for selection of points and references for treatment. Diseases discussed here include internal diseases, surgical diseases, gynecological diseases, pediatric diseases, and diseases of the eye, ear, nose, throat and mouth cavity. Besides, there is schematic diagram for the selection of points attached to each disease to facilitate the reader's use.

Based on clinical practice, this book deals with a wide range of diseases with combined use of words and illustrations. Being easy to understand and very practical, this book can be a reference for professionals and other medical workers and those who are interested in auricular-point-pressing therapy.

Shan Qiuhua
Jinan
P. R. China

Contents

Introduction

Auricular-point-pressing therapy is a therapeutic method in which plant seeds with hard texture and smooth surface, or prepared medicines with a suitable shape and texture are pressed on auricular points with plaster tape to treat diseases. It is now the most extensively used method for stimulating auricular points, and also a simple alternative for auricular needle-embedding.

I. Mechanism of Auricular-Point-Pressing Therapy

1. The theory of Zang-Fu organs and Meridians

Explanation of the mechanism of using auricular points to treat diseases of the whole body can be dated back to *Nei Jing* (*Internal Classic of Medicine*). The book states that the ear is very closely related to meridians. The chapter *Xie Qi Zang Fu Bing Xing Pian* (*Manifestation of Pathogenic Factors and Zang-Fu Organs*) of *Ling Shu* (*Miraculous Pivot*) states that Blood and Qi in the twelve Channels and three hundred and sixty-five Collaterals run upwards to the face and then enter the orifices... the rest of the Qi enters the ear to support hearing ability. The chapter *Jing Mai* (*Meridians*) of *Ling*

Shu (*Miraculous Pivot*) describes the distribution of six Yang Channels in the ear:

One branch of the Small Intestine Channel of Hand-Taiyang enters the ear.

One branch of the Sanjiao Channel of Hand-Shaoyang originates behind the ear and runs upwards along the posterior border of the ear to enter the superior aspect of the ear, and the other branch arises from the retro- auricular region, enters the ear, and then emerges in front of the ear.

One branch of the gallbladder Channel of Foot-Shaoyang runs from the retro-auricular region to the ear and then emerges in front of the ear.

The divergent Channel of Hand-Yangming enters the ear and joins the Assembled Channel (Zong Mai).

The Stomach Channel of Foot-Yangming ascends to the preauricular region.

One branch of the Bladder Channel of Foot-Taiyang splits off the vertex of the head and descends to the upper aspect of the auricle.

The Chapter *Jing Jin* (*Muscle Regions*) of *Ling Shu* (*Miraculous Pivot*) describes the connections between the ear and the muscle region of the Foot-Yangming, Hand-Taiyang and Hand-Shaoyang. According to *Ling Shu* (*Miraculous Pivot*), three Yang Channels of the hand and the foot have the most close connections with the auricular region. The six Yin Channels associate with the Yang Channels via *Jing Bie* (*Divergent Channels*) though they do not connect the ear directly. Therefore, all the twelve regular Channels run to the ear directly or indirectly. Hence the chapter *Kou Wen* (*Question*) of *Ling Shu* (*Miraculous Pivot*) says that the ear is the assembled place of Channels. Considerable modern experiments have showed that there are Channels and Collaterals existing in the auricle, which connect with meridians of the whole body. For example, stimulating the auricular point can elicit propagated sensation along the corresponding Channel. The propagated sensation usually originates from the ear and runs along a certain course to the starting or terminating point of the corresponding Channel, and then transmits along the Channel. Up to now, numerous clinical observations and experimental studies have been conducted by means of Channel transmission, synthermal spectrum analysis, auricular staining method, radioisotope tracing method, etc. Achievements have preliminarily confirmed that the auricle has Channel transmission relation with the internal organs, the five sense organs and the body points. The auricular meridians are a connecting part of the whole Channel system, which is the basis for the fact that pressing at the auricle can treat diseases in the remote part of the body.

In addition to Channels, the ear is also very closely related with Zang-Fu organs. The chapter *Wu Yue Wu Shi* (*Five Zang Organs and Their Corresponding Manifestations*) of *Ling Shu* (*Miraculous Pivot*) says the ear is the orifice of the Kidney. The chapter *Mai Du* (*Measurement of Meridians*) of *Ling Shu* (*Miraculous Pivot*) says the Kidney Qi connects with the ear, therefore, a sound Kidney is the basis for the hearing of the ear. The chapter *Jin Gui Zhen Yan Lun* (*Maxim of Golden Chamber*) of *Su Wen* (*Plain Questions*) says the ear connects with the Heart. The chapter *Zang Qi Fa Shi Lun* (*Internal Organs Following the Example of Climate*) of *Su Wen* (*Plain Questions*) says that deficiency of the Liver brings about loss of hearing, and adverse flow of the Liver Qi causes headache and deafness. The chapter *Yu Ji Zhen Zang Lun* (*Mystery of Zang Organs*) of *Su Wen* (*Plain Questions*) says dysfunction of the Spleen causes obstruction of the nine orifices. *Si Shi Nan* (*The Fortieth Difficulty*) of *Nan Jing* (*Classic of Difficulties*) says that the Lung controls voice and enables the ear to hear. Zhang Zhenjun, a physician in the Qing Dynasty, collected the experiences recorded in ancient medical works and put forward a theory of distribution of five Zang organs on the auricle. From the above explanation, we can see that the ear is very closely related with the physiological function of the viscera and bowels which has been confirmed by experimental research and clinical practice. For example, disorder of internal organs may reflex itself on the corresponding points of the auricle, such as low electrical resistance and tender spot. And stimulating those reaction points with needling or pressing can improve symptoms or cure disease. Those reaction may reduce or disappear along with the improvement of the diseased organs or recovery of disease.

2. The theory of Neurohumor

The auricle is richly supplied by nerves which include great auricular nerve and lesser occipital nerve deriving from the plexus of the spinal nerve, auriculotemporal nerve deriving from the cranial nerve, and branches from the facial nerve, glossopharyngeal nerve, vagus nerve and sympathetic nerve. Besides, the auricle skin contains a variety of neuroreceptors, such as free sensory nerve endings, follocular sensory nerve endings and corpuscula lamellosa. In the tendon and muscle of the auricle, there are plexiform sensory nerve endings both simple and complex, Golgi tendon organs, Ruffini's nerve endings and muscular spindles. Therefore, the auricular points are highly sensitive to various stimuli.

When a disease occurs, the pathological impulse connects with the corresponding neurons and greatly improves their excitability, which in turn will affect the sensation threshold of the auricular points projecting on these neurons or those nearby, and then improves the sensitivity. The optical stimulation resulting from treatments brings about an ecological inhibition on the respective neurons by retarding the former pathological afferent impulse, or producing a strong excitability which inhibits the original pathological excitability of the adjacent neurons according to the preferential principle. In this way, the vicious cycle of pathological impulse is blocked, the orientation of the pathological interchange of cause and effect is changed, while a pathological regulation takes place instead and leads to the improvement or recovery of the disease.

According to modern medicine, the inseparable relation among all parts of the body and all functions of the body is ensured by the combined neurohumoral regulation. Therefore, this regulation is considered by some physicians to play an important role in the mechanism of ear acupuncture. Through the neurohumoral system, an favorable stimulation produces effects on dynamic equilibrium of the body and makes the immuno-defensive system work positively, thus a disease is cured.

3. The theory of Embryo Complete Information of Wholistic Organ (ECIWO)

ECIWO was proposed by Professor Zhang Yingqing in 1973. At the beginning, he found that the second metacarpal bond seems exactly to be a miniature of the whole body. Whether or not there is tender spot on the radial side and where the location of the tender spot is can tell us whether or not there is disorder in the body and where the focus of the disorder is. And needling or massage at the tender spot can treat diseases occurring in the corresponding area. Professor Zhang points out that any relatively independent part of the body has the same regularity of point distribution as the second metacarpal bone.

In the·1950's, Nogier, a Frenchman, put forward an "inverted-fetus like" distribution of auricular points. According to this law, each of the Five Zang organs, Six Fu organs, four limbs and all bones, five sense organs, even a much smaller part of the body has its corresponding location on the auricle, which looks like a miniature fetus twisted inside the uterus with its head down and buttock up. This distribution law of auricular points conforms with the ECIWO. Therefore, the ECIWO is considered to be a theoretical basis for auricular therapy.

According to ECIWO, the auricle, as a relatively isolated part of the body, is a miniature of the whole body and contains all the information the body possesses. Based on this viewpoint, a ECIWO reflex was proposed to explain the transmission mechanism of the auricular information. According to the doctrine, the ECIWO reflex center formed by ECIWO-related neurons forms a reflex pathway. Thc ECWIO relation of the cerebral neurons refers to the dual-directional synaptic relation between the two projections on the nerve center, one from the representative region of any relatively independent part of the body, the other from the corresponding part of the organism. It is through this relation that the information transmission is carried on between the auricular point and its corresponding part of the body.

The mechanism of ECIWO explains the direct connection between the focus and the auricular reaction area, that is, one focus has only one auricular reaction area. However, it is a fact that one disease reflexes itself on many auricular points. To answer this, the integral whole and coordination of organic body should be taken into account. As an organic whole, all the organs and systems of the body function cooperatively instead of separately. When one organ is diseased, the tissues and organs closely related to it are often affected, which will manifest themselves on the corresponding auricular points when they develop to a certain degree. Therefore, one disease may have positive reactions in several auricular points. Stimulating these points can produce influences on their corresponding parts of the body.

Ⅱ. Characteristics of Auricular-point-pressing Therapy

Auricular-point-pressing therapy is developed from auricular needling. It possesses the advantages of being easy to learn, simple, convenient, safe and practical to use, having wide indications, reliable therapeutic effects and few side effects.

1. Easy to learn, simple and convenient to use

Since auricular points have a regular distribution and most of them are named after internal organs and anatomic sites, those with certain knowledge of both TCM and Western medicine can master it after a short- term study. International standardization of auricular points makes it easier for clinical workers to learn and use.

Instead of special equipment, auricular-point-pressing therapy can be performed with some simple materials, such as 75% alcohol cotton ball, hard medicinal pill, plant or specially-made seeds, medical adhesive plaster, and forceps. It can be applied anytime and anywhere, without regard to surroundings and posture of the patient. The patient can move about freely during the period of treatment and can perform stimulation on points under the instruction of the doctor. Therefore, it is welcomed by both clinicians and patients.

2. Wide indications and reliable effects

Auricular-point-pressing can be used not only for treatment but also for prevention, health preservation and improvement of looks. According to statistics, it has been applied for treatment of more than one hundred diseases including internal diseases, surgical diseases, gynecological diseases, pediatric diseases and diseases of the eye, ear, nose, throat and mouth. This therapy is effective against diseases, especially acute inflammation and pain syndromes. For example, biliary colic, toothache and sprain can be relieved or stopped within several minutes after auricular therapy is given. The sleep of a patient suffering from neurosism can be improved 1—2 days after the treatment starts. Ding Yude etal has reported that the effective rate of auricular-point-pressing was 93.98%, 97.62% and 97.77% respectively in treating internal diseases, surgical diseases and other kinds of diseases such as diseases of dermatology, eye, ear, nose, throat and gynecology. In addition, auricular point-pressing has preventive effects for the common cold, acute conjunctivitis, mumps and transfusion reaction.

3. Safe and practical with few side effects

Auricular-point-pressing causes little suffering and few side effects and has no such toxic and adverse effects as drugs. Since it will not damage tissues and organs, inflammation and infection due to improper sterilization are avoided. Besides, auricular therapy produces a persistent stimulation and a stable therapeutic efficacy. Therefore, it is very easily accepted by patients. Auricular-point-pressing is especially suitable for those who are old, very young, generally weak, nervous or afraid of needling.

Anatomy of the Auricle

Auricle is formed by elastic cartilage, cartilage membrane, ligament, degenerative auricular muscle, subcutaneous tissues and skin. The subcutaneous tissues are rich in nerves, vessels and lymph. The ear lobe is formed by fat and connective tissues without cartilage.

I. Anatomical Areas of the Auricular Surface

1. Anatomical areas of the anterior auricular surface (Fig. 2—1)

Helix: The curling rim of the most lateral border of the auricle.

Helix tubercle: A small tubercle at the lateral-superior aspect of the helix.

End of Helix: The lowest border of the helix connecting with the ear lobe.

Root of helix (Helix crus): A transverse ridge of the helix continuing backward into the ear cavity.

Antihelix: At the medial aspect of the helix, the protruding curving ridge parallel to the helix.

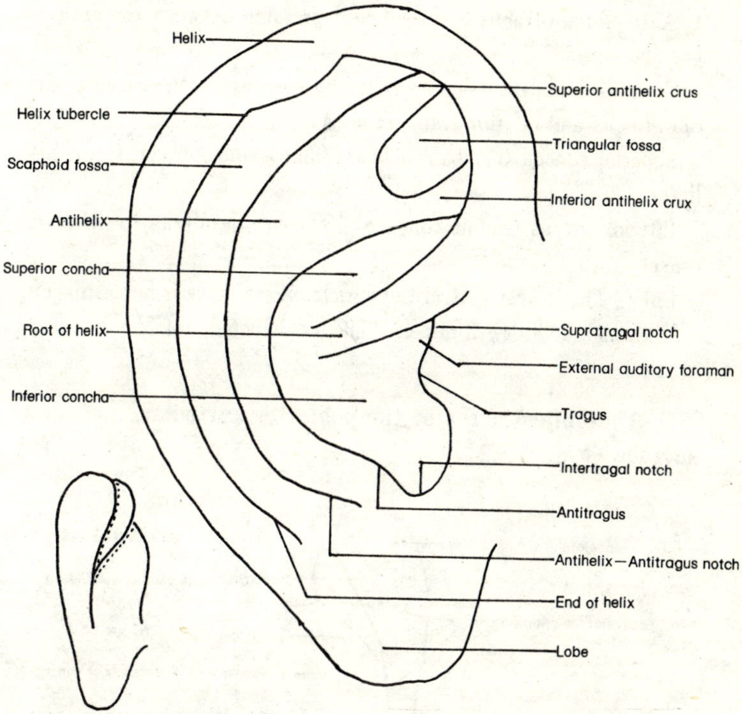

Fig. 2—1 Anatomical areas of anterior surface of auricle

Superior antihelix crus: The upper branch of the antihelix.

Inferior antihelix crus: The lower branch of the antihelix.

Triangular fossa: The triangular depression between the two crura of the antihelix.

Scaphoid fossa: The narrow curved depression between the helix and the antihelix.

Tragus: A curved flap in front of the auricle.

Antitragus: A small tubercle opposite to the tragus and superior to the upper part of the ear lobe.

Supratragal notch: The depression between the upper border of the tragus and the helix crus.

Intertragal notch: The depression between the tragus and the antitragus.

Antihelix-antitragus notch: The depression between the antitragus and antihelix.

Concha: The depression encircled by antitragus, the curving part of antihelix and inferior antihelix crus.

Superior concha (cymba conchae): The cavum superior to the helix crus.

Inferior concha (cavum conchae): The cavum inferior to the helix crus.

Lobe: The lowest part of the auricle where there is no cartilage.

External auditory foramen: The out opening of the auditory canal.

2. Anatomical areas of the posterior auricular surface (Fig. 2—2)

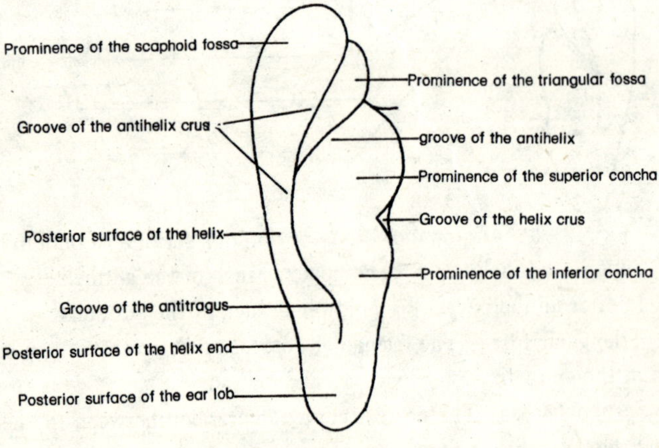

Fig. 2—2 Anatomical areas of posterior surface of auricle

There are three flat areas, four grooves and four protruding parts in the posterior auricular surface.

Posterior surface of the helix: Lateral aspect of the helix. Since the helix curves forwards, the aspect faces ahead.

Posterior surface of the helix end: The flat area between the posterior surfaces of the scaphoid fossa and the ear lobe.

Posterior surface of the ear lobe: The flat area of the ear lobe.

Groove of the antihelix: The groove in the posterior surfaces of the antihelix crus and antihelix body.

Groove of the antihelix crus: The depression in the posterior surface of the antihelix, running from the interior to the exterior. It is also called upper groove of the posterior surface.

Groove of the helix crus: The posterior surface of the helix crus.

Groove of the antitragus: The posterior surface of the antitragus.

Prominence of the scaphoid fossa: The prominence of the posterior surface of the scaphoid fossa.

Prominence of the triangular fossa: The posterior surface of the triangular fossa, e.g. the prominence between the groove of the superior antihelix crus and the groove of the inferior antihelix crus.

Prominence of the superior concha: The prominence of the posterior surface of the superior concha.

Prominence of the inferior concha: The prominence of the posterior surface of the inferior concha.

Ⅱ. Blood Vessel Distribution of the Auricle

1. Artery

The superficial temporal artery and posterior auricular artery, which derive from the external carotid artery, run along the perichondrium in the deep lay of the auricle.

The superficial temporal artery branches 3—4 rami auriculares anteriores which are distributed in the anterior part of the anterior aspect. Posterior auricular artery ascends along the root of the auricle and separates several rami auriculares anteriores which are distributed in the posterior surface of the auricle. The posterior auricular artery also splits several penetrating branches which penetrate the helix, triangular fossa and superior concha to the anterior aspect of the auricle, and a rami auriculares anterior which passes through the lower margin of the cartilage and then is distributed in the helix, scaphoid fossa and antihelix.

There are rather large anastomonic branches between the superficial temporal artery, the posterior auricular artery and the occipital artery, which connect the anterior and the posterior. Since all these arteries are separated in the root of the auricle or external auditory foramen and run to the lateral rim of the auricle, the skin temperature of auricular point proximal to the root of the ear is higher than those distal to it.

2. Vein

The veins usually accompany with the artery. In the anterior surface of the auricle, veins are somewhat smaller and located in a more shallow lay than arteries. In triangular fossa, veins form venous network. Many of the anterior auricular veins run forwards and directly pour into the superficial temporal vein. Veins from the helix, the scaphoid fossa and the ear lobe converge into a large one, the rami auriculares anteriores of the posterior auricular vein, which pours into the posterior auricular vein in the posterior surface of the auricle after passing the lower margin of the cartilage. All the veins in the posterior aspect of the auricle converge into 3－5 rami auriculares posteriores, which run transversely towards the root of the ear and join the posterior auricular vein.

Ⅲ. Nerve Distribution of the Auricle

The auricle is richly supplied by nerves. The nerves include the somatic nerves which derive from the great auricular nerve and lesser occipital nerve, the cranial nerves such as the branches from the auriculotemporal nerve, facial nerve, lingual nerve and vagus nerve and sympathetic nerve.

Great auricular nerve derives from the cervical plexus (C2—3) at the midway of the posterior margin of the sternocleidomastoid muscle. It curves to the surface of the muscle and branches the rema auriculares anteriores and the rema auriculares posteriores at the same level as the ear lobe. The former crosses the ear lobe to the anterior aspect of the auricle, ascends along the scaphoid fossa and supplies the ear lobe, the helix, the antihelix, the lower 2/3 portion of the scaphoid fossa, the antitragus, the superior concha, the lateral part of inferior concha and the posterior part of the triangular fossa. The latter supplies the lower 2/3 portion of the posterior aspect of the auricle.

Lesser occipital nerve also derives from the cervical plexus (C2) and runs upwards along the posterior margin of the sternocleidomastoid muscle. It branches rema auriculares anteriores and perforating branches which supply the helix, the upper part of scaphoid fossa, the superior antihelix crus and part of the triangular fossa. Its rema auriculares posteriores supply the upper 1/3 portion of the posterior aspect of the auricle.

The auricular branch of the vagus nerve derives from the jugular neuroganglion; it is in fact the peripheral synapse of the pseudounipolar neuron in the neuroganglion. Running forwards and passing through the lateral wall of the jugular fossa, it enters the facial canal and meets with the facial nerve trunk there. Going out of the stylomastoid foramen, it departs from the facial nerve trunk and ascends along the posterior groove of the auricle and surface of the mastoid during which it splits several small branches which are distributed in the posterior aspect of the auricle, and perforating branches as well, to the anterior aspect of the auricle.

The posterior auricular nerve splits from the facial nerve after the nerve runs out of the stylomastoid foramen. It ascends upwards along the posterior groove of the auricle. In the retro-auricular region, it branches the posterior auricular branch to control the posterior auricular muscle and occipital muscle. It also splits an anterior perforating branch to the anterior aspect of the auricle.

Fiber-exchange may exist between the anterior perforating branch of the vagus nerve and the anterior perforating branch of the posterior auricular nerve of the facial nerve. They all penetrate the auricular cartilage and are distributed in the superior concha, inferior concha, external auditory canal, helix crus and triangular fossa. There are anastomotic branches between the glossopharyngeal nerve and the vagus nerve, which are distributed along with the vagus nerve.

The sympathetic nerve derives from the carotid plexus. It is distributed along the artery. The density of the nervous fibers are reduced with the decrease of the artery caliber, a few in the vein and the most in the anastomotic branch. There are crisscross fibers between the artery and the vein.

In conclusion, in the anterior aspect of the auricle, the great auricular nerve supplies the ear lobe, the helix, the scaphoid fossa, the antihelix, the antitragus, the superior concha, the inferior concha and lateral part of the triangular fossa; the lesser occipital nerve supplies the upper edge of the auricle; the auricular temporal nerve supplies the tragus, the helix crus and the internal part of the ear lobe, the superior concha and the triangular fossa; and the rema auriculares posteriores of the facial nerve and the auricular branch of the vagus never supply the superior concha, the inferior concha and the triangular fossa. In the posterior aspect of the auricle, the lesser occipital nerve supplies the upper 1/3 portion while the great auricular nerve supplies the lower 2/3 portions.

Ⅳ. Lymph Distribution of the Auricle

The auricle is also richly supplied by lymphatic vessels. The lymph vessels are net-like and the lymph flows into the lymph nodes in the vicinity of the auricle. According to the flow direction of the lymph, the lymph vessels are divided into three groups: the anterior, the posterior and the inferior.

The anterior group: It includes the lymph vessels in the anterior aspect of the auricle and the upper wall of the auditory canal. The lymph flows into the lymphoglandulae auriculares anteriores and the parotid lymph node.

The posterior group: It refers to the lymph vessels in the posterior aspect of the auricle. The lymph drains into the lymphoglandulae retroauricular lymph nodes.

The lower group: It includes the lymph vessels in the ear lobe and the lower wall of the external auditory canal. The lymph drains into the retroauricular nodes.

All lymph of the above three groups drain into the deep cervical lymph nodes and finally into the venous angle.

V. Cartilage and Muscle of the Auricle

The muscles of the auricle include the intra-auricular muscles , which attach the auricular cartilage, and the external auricular muscles, which attach the auricle and the ranial bone.

The intra-auricular muscles: They include the great muscle of helix, smaller muscle of helix, tragus muscle, antitragus muscle, transverse muscle of auricle and oblique muscle of auricle.

External auricular muscles: They include superior auricular muscle, posterior auricular muscle and anterior auricular muscle.

Apart from a few individuals whose external auricular muscle has contractive function to move the auricle, for most people, the function of the auricular muscles have degenerated and only left some traces. In a perspective of histology, the degenerated auricular muscles are found in locations of many auricular points such as Kidney (MA—SC), Bladder (MA—SC8), Occiput (MA—AT), Groove of Posterior Auricle (MA—PS) and Upper Ear Root (MA—PS).

Auricular cartilage: Except the ear lobe, the whole auricle is supported by cartilage.

Auricular Points

I . Definition and Distributive Regularity of Auricular Points

1. Definition

Auricular points are the sites where the auricle links with the Zang and Fu organs, Channels and Collaterals, tissues and organs, four limbs and all bones. They are also the points through which the Channel Qi (Jing Qi) is transported to the auricle. Therefore, the spots on the auricle where physiological functions and pathological changes can be reflected are called auricular points, which are the specific spots used for diagnosis and treatment of disease.

When the internal organs or part of the body is in an abnormal condition, various positive reactions will appear in the corresponding area of the auricle. Therefore, by analysis of changes of these positive reaction points, we can deduce the location and nature of a disease and, furthermore, treat the disease by applying various stimulation to these auricular points. Auricular points are often called reaction points, sensitive points, positive points, tender points, lower resistance points, high conductivity points, or treatment points.

2. Distributive regularity

Auricular points are distributed regularly on the auricle. On the anterior-lateral surface, the distribution of auricular points is just like an inverted fetus in the womb, with the head downwards, buttocks and legs upwards, and chest and trunk in the middle. The distributive regularity is as follows:

Points located on the antitragus and lobe are related to the head and facial region, those in the scaphoid fossa to the upper limbs, those at the antihelix to the trunk, those at the superior and inferior antihelix crus to the lower limbs and buttocks, those in the triangular fossa to the pelvis, those around the helix to the digestive tract, those in the superior concha to the abdominal cavity, those in the inferior concha to the thoracic cavity, those at the tragus to the nasopharynx, and those at the intertragus notch to the endocrine.

Ⅱ. Nomenclature of Auricular Points

Sun Simiao, a famous medical expert of the Tang Dynasty, said in his works *Qian Jin Yao Fang* (*Thousand Ducat Prescriptions*) that each point has a corresponding name with a profound implication. This is to say that the name of an auricular point has a specific meaning. Therefore, learning the nomenclature of points can help memorize and understand their clinical applications. The nomenclature of auricular points is summarized as follows.

1. According to anatomical area

This is the basic way in which points are named according to the projection of an anatomical area on the auricle. For example, the scaphoid fossa is the projection of the upper limbs, so points located in the scaphoid are named Shoulder (MA－SF4), Elbow (MA－SF3), Wrist (MA－SF2), Finger (MA－SF1) and so on. The area around the helix crus is the projection of digestive tract, so points here are named Mouth (MA—IC5), Esophagus (MA—IC6), Cardia (MA—IC7), Stomach (MA—IC), Duodenum (MA—SC1), Small Intestine (MA—SC2), Appendix (MA—SC3), Large Intestine (MA—SC4), etc.

2. According to the theory of Zang-Fu organs and Meridians

Auricular points are named after Zang-Fu organs and Meridians according to the focus of disease and the regularity of treatment, such as Heart (MA—IC), Liver (MA—SC5), Spleen (MA—IC), Lung (MA—IC1), Kidney (MA—SC), Bladder (MA—SC8) and Sanjiao (NA—IC4). The name of these points indicates some content of the theory of Zang-Fu organs and Meridians. For example, Heart (MA—IC) can be a positive reaction spot of the Heart disorder and sore and insomnia as well, and it has proven effective for treatment of these disorders. This is the embodiment of the Heart controlling Blood and Vessels and taking charge of mental activities according to the theory of Zang-Fu organs.

3. According to functions of auricular points

Auricular points are named according to their functions in both TCM and Western medicine.

From the perspective of TCM, Wind Stream (MA—SF) and Shenmen (MA—TF1) are named because Wind Stream (MA—SF) has the function of dispelling Wind and relieving itching and is often used to treat urticaria and cutaneous pruritis while Shenmen (MA—TF1) has the function of tranquilizing the mind, regulating mental activities and hypnotizing and is often used to treat insomnia, dream-disturbed sleep and pain syndromes.

From the perspective of Western medicine, Sympathetic (MA—AH7) is named since it has the similar functions to the vegetative nerve and is effective against dysfunction of the vegetative nerve, internal organs and glands. Adrenal Gland (MA—T) is named because it has the similar function to adrenaline such as elevating blood pressure and antianaphylaxix. And Endocrine (MA—IC3) is named since it has the function of regulating endocrine.

4. According to numerical order

In this way, Eye1 (MA—L), Eye (MA—L), Tumor-distinctive Area1,2,3, (MA) etc. are named.

The nomenclature of auricular points is generalized as the above four ways. However, for a certain point, its nomenclature may not be simply classified into one approach. For example, nomenclature of Lung (MA—IC1) and Heart (MA—IC) is based on both anatomical area and the theory of Zang-Fu organs and Meridians. Sympathetic (MA—AH7) derives its name from both its function and neuroanatomy. Therefore, to select points appropriately and to obtain satisfactory therapeutic results, one should understand the meaning of a point comprehensively.

Ⅲ. Nomenclature, Location, Function and Indicatio of the Standardized Auricular Points

The number of auricular points is more than 300 according to incomplete statistics. Auricular therapy is applied in about 100 countries in the world. However, the nomenclature and location are not unified. To facilitate international exchange, it is necessary to standardize this ancient diagnostic and therapeutic method. In 1986, All-China Association of Acupuncture and Moxibustion was empowered by the WHO Regional Office for the Western Pacific to lay down a draft The Scheme of International Standardization of Auricular Points. About ninety points are adopted in this scheme. In June from 25th to 30th, 1987, WHO Regional Office for the Western Pacific held the Third WHO Regional Working Group meeting on the Standardization of Acupuncture Nomenclature in Seoul. On the basis of Chinese scheme of auricular points, Seventy-nine points out of

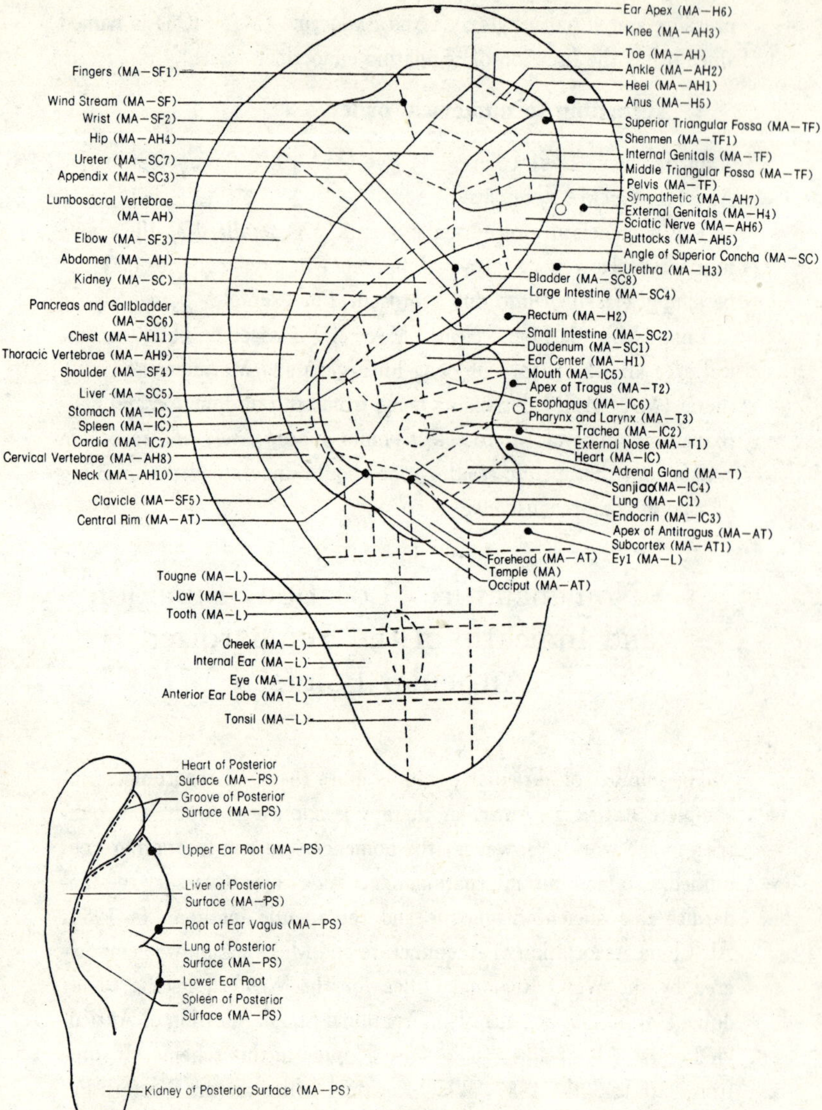

Fig. 3－1 Auricular points adopted by the WHO Regional office for the Pacific (1987)

the ninety points originally presented were adopted (Fig. 3—1). Among the seventy-nine points, forty-three points have the same name and location in both Chinese and French auricular points, which are named with proper coding; thirty-six points have the same name but different locations, which are not given the coding, and the remaining eleven points were not accepted. Based on the Chinese scheme, the name, location, function and indication of auricular points are described as follows.

1. The helix points (Fig. 3—2)

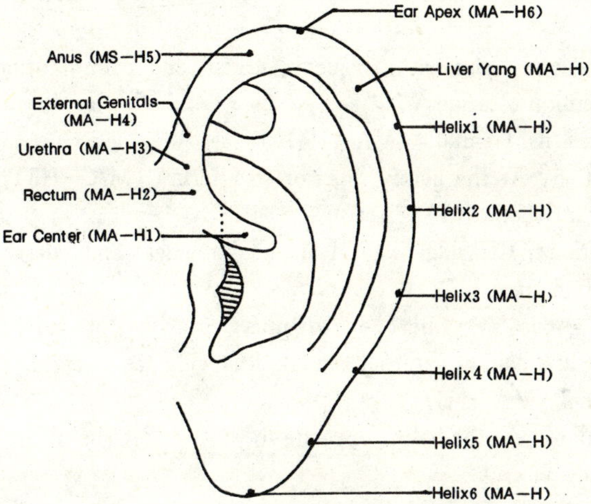

Fig. 3—2 The helix points

1) Middle Ear (MA—H1) (former name: Zero Point, Diaphragm, Neurosism Point)

Location: On the helix crus.

Functions: Sending down adverse flow of Qi and normalizing the function of diaphragm, regulating Blood, and dispelling Wind.

Indications: Hiccup, urticaria, skin itching, infantile enuresis, hemoptysis, and epistaxis.

2) Rectum (MA—H2) (former name: Lower Rectum)

Location: At the helix near supratragus notch, level with Large Intestine (MA—SC4).

Functions: Invigorating Qi and regulating Intestines, relaxing bowels or checking diarrhea, and relieving inflammation and pain.

Indications: Prolapse of anus, constipation or diarrhea, and hemorrhoids.

3) Urethra (MA—H3)

Location: At the helix, superior to Rectum (MA—H2), level with Bladder (MA—SC8).

Functions: Relieving inflammation and pain and promoting urination.

Indications: Enuresis, frequent, urgent and painful urination, and retention of urine.

4) External Genitalia (MA—H4)

Location: At the helix, superior to Urethra (MA—H3), level with Sympathetic (MA—AH7).

Functions: Clearing away Heat and Dampness and relieving inflammation and pain.

Indications: Orchitis, epididymitis, pruritus of vulva, and swelling and pain of external genitals following vasoligation.

5) Anus (MA—H5)

Locations: At the helix, opposite to the anterior rim of the superior antihelix crus.

Functions: Relieving inflammation and pain.

Indications: Hemorrhoids and anal fissure.

6) Ear Apex (MA—H6)

Location: At the top of the helix, opposite to the posterior border of the superior antihelix crus.

Functions: Clearing away Heat and Toxic Materials, calming the Liver, depressing Wind, and relieving inflammation and pain.

Indications: Fever, hypertension, acute conjunctivitis and hordeolum, acne, and acute tonsillitis.

7) Liver Yang (MA—H)

Location: At the helix tubercle.

Functions: Clearing away Heat and Toxic Materials, calming the Liver and suppressing the hyperactivity of Yang.

Indications: Dizziness, headache and hypertension, and swelling and pain of the eye and hepatalgia.

8) Helix 1—6 (MA—H)

Location: Divide the helix area into five equal parts from the lower border of the helix tubercle to the midpoint of the lower border of the ear lobe. The points making the divisions are respectively named Helix 1, 2, 3, 4, 5 and 6.

Functions: Clearing away Heat and Toxic Materials and relieving swelling and pain.

Indications: Tonsillitis, infections of the upper respiratory tract, and fever.

2. The scaphoid fossa points (Fig. 3—3)

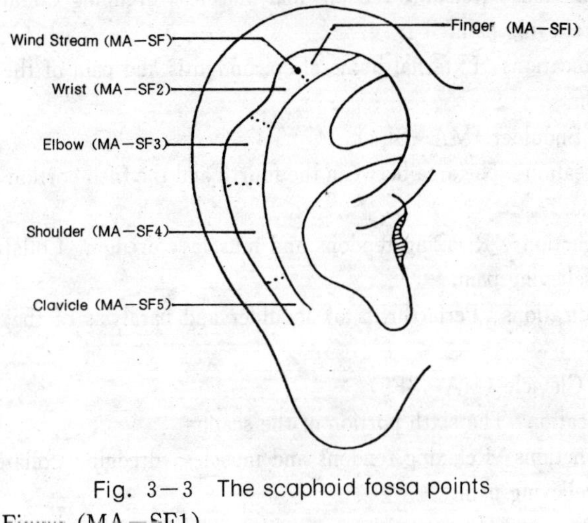

Fig. 3—3 The scaphoid fossa points

1) Finger (MA—SF1)

Location: Divide the scapha into six portions from upward to downward, the first portion is Finger (MA—SF1).

Functions: Relieving inflammation, dredging Collaterals, and stopping pain.

Indications: Paronychia and pain and numbness of fingers.

2) Wind Stream (MA—SF)

Location: In the scapha, at the midpoint between Finger (MA—SF1) and Wrist (MA—SF2).

Functions: Dispelling Wind, arresting itching, relieving cough and asthma, and checking allergic reaction.

Indications: Urticaria, cutaneous pruritus, asthma, and allergic rhinitis.

3) Wrist (MA—SF2)

Location: The second portion of the scapha.

Functions: Relaxing tendons and muscles, dredging Collaterals, and relieving pain.

Indications: Pain of the wrist region.

4) Elbow (MA—SF3)

Location: The third portion of the scapha.

Functions: Relaxing tendons and muscles, dredging Collaterals, and relieving pain.

Indications: External humeral epicondylitis and pain of the wrist region.

5) Shoulder (MA—SF4)

Location: The area between the fourth and the fifth portion of the scapha.

Functions: Relaxing tendons and muscles, dredging Collaterals, and relieving pain.

Indications: Periarthritis of shoulder and paralysis of the upper limb.

6) Clavicle (MA—SF5)

Location: The sixth portion of the scapha.

Functions: Relaxing tendons and muscles, dredging Collaterals, and relieving pain.

Indications: Periarthritis of shoulder and pain of the neck and upper back.

3. The antihelix points (Fig. 3—4)

1) Toe (MA—AH)

Location: At the posterior and superior corner of the superior antihelix crus, near the ear apex.

Functions: Relaxing tendons and muscles, activating Blood, and relieving swelling and pain.

Indications: Paronychia and pain of the toes, Raynaud's disease, and erythromelalgia.

2) Heel (MA—AH1)

Location: At the anterior and superior corner of the superior antihelix crus, near upper end of the triangular fossa.

Functions: Relaxing tendons and muscles, strengthening bones, and relieving swelling and pain.

Indications: Heel pain.

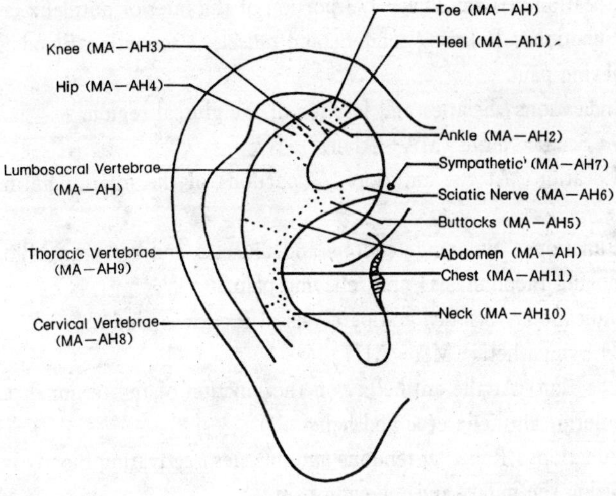

Fig. 3—4 The antihelix points

3) Ankle (MA—SH2)

Location: Midway between Heel (MA—AH1) and Knee (MA—AH3).

Functions: Relaxing tendons and muscles, activating Blood, and relieving pain.

Indications: Sprain and contusion of ankle joint.

4) Knee (MA—AH3)

Location: At the middle 1/3 portion of the superior antihelix crus.

Functions: Dispelling Wind and activating Blood, dredging Collaterals, and relieving pain.

Indications: Swelling and pain of knee joint and rheumatic arthritis.

5) Hip (MA—AH4)

Location: At the lower 1/3 portion of the superior antihelix crus

Functions: Relaxing tendons and muscles, activating Blood, and relieving pain.

Indications: Pain of the hip joint and sciatica.

6) Buttocks (MA—AH5)

Location: At the lower 1/3 portion of the inferior antihelix crus.

Functions: Relaxing tendons and muscles, activating Blood, and relieving pain.

Indications: Sciatica and fasciitis of the gluteal region.

7) Sciatic Nerve (MA—AH6)

Location: At the anterior 2/3 portions of the inferior antihelix crus.

Functions: Relaxing tendons and muscles and activating Blood, removing Blood stasis, and relieving pain.

Indications: Sciatica and paralysis of the lower limb.

8) Sympathetic (MA—AH7)

Location: At the antihelix, on the junction of the terminal point of inferior antihelix crus and helix.

Functions: Relaxing tendons and muscles, activating Blood, tranquilizing the mind, and relieving pain.

Indications: Gastrointestinal spasm, angina pectoris, biliary colic, calculi of ureter, dysfunction of the autonomous nervous system, acrotism, and asthma.

9) Cervical Vertebrae (MA—AH8)

Location: A curved line from the helix-tragic notch to the bifurcation of the superior and inferior antihelix crura is divided into five equal segments. The lower 1/5 portion of it is the cervical vertebrae (MA—AH 8), the middle 2/5 is thoracic vertebrae (MA—AH 9) and the upper 2/5 is the lumbosacral vertebrae (MA—AH).

Functions: Relaxing tendons and muscles and activating Blood, strengthening bones, dredging Collaterals, and relieving pain.

Indications: Stiffneck and cervical spondylopathy.

10) Thoracic Vertebrae (MA—AH9)

Location: At the middle 2/5 of the antihelix.

Functions: Relaxing tendons and muscles, nourishing Marrow, dredging Collaterals, and relieving pain.

Indications: Pain in the thoracic and hypochondriums, mastitis, insufficient lactation, ankylosing spondylitis, premenstrual mammary distension and pain, mastitis, and oligogalactia.

11) Lumbosacral Vertebrae (MA—AH)

Location: At the upper 2/5 of the antihelix.

Functions: Strengthening the loins and replenishing the Kidney, dredging Collaterals, and relieving pain.

Indications: Pain at the lumbosacral area.

12) Neck (MA—AH10)

Location: At the lower part of the antihelix, at the anterior aspect of Cervical Vertebrae (MA—AH8), near the rim of scapha.

Functions: Relaxing tendons and muscles, dredging Collaterals, and relieving inflammation and pain.

Indications: Stiffneck and swelling and pain of the neck.

13) Chest (MA—AH11)

Location: At the middle part of the antihelix, at the anterior aspect of Thoracic Vertebrae (MA—AH9), near the rim of scapha.

Functions: Regulating the flow of Qi and alleviating depression, and relieving inflammation and pain.

Indications: Fullness of the chest, hypochondriac pain, and mastitis.

14) Abdomen (MA—AH)

Location: At the upper part of thc antihclix, at the anterior aspect of Lumbosacral Vertebrae (MA—AH), near the rim of scapha.

Functions: Strengthening the Spleen and the Stomach, dredging Collaterals, and relieving pain.

Indications: Abdominal pain and distension, diarrhea, and acute sprain.

4. The triangular fossa points (Fig. 3—5)

1) Shenmen (MA—TF1)

Location: In the triangular fossa, at the superior aspect of the bifurcating point between the superior and the inferior antihelix crura.

Functions: Calming the Heart and tranquilizing the mind, relieving spasm and pain, and alleviating inflammation and itching.

Indications: Insomnia, dream-disturbed sleep, pain syndrome, withdrawal syndrome, urticaria, pruritis, and asthma.

2) Pelvis (MA—TF) (former name: Lumbago Point)

Location: In the triangular fossa, slightly inferior to the medial side of the bifurcating point between the superior and the inferior antihelix crura.

Functions: Dredging Collaterals and activating Blood, relieving inflammation, and stopping pain.

Indications: Pelvic inflammation.

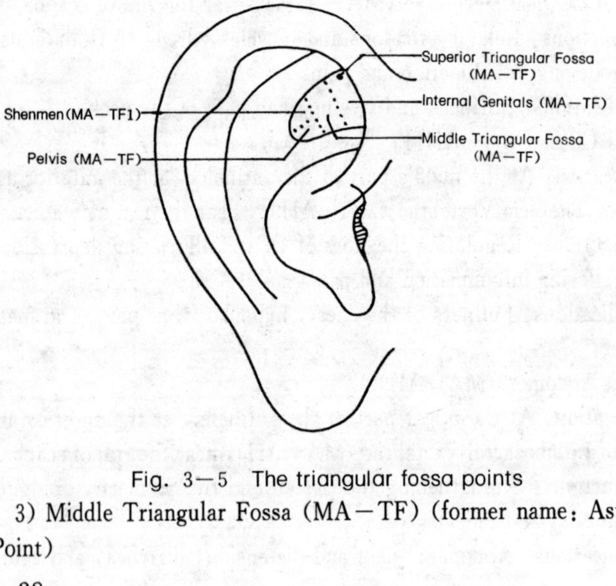

Fig. 3—5 The triangular fossa points

3) Middle Triangular Fossa (MA—TF) (former name: Asthma Point)

Location: In the middle 1/3 of the triangular fossa.

Functions: Relieving cough and asthma, soothing the Liver Qi, and promoting the function of the Gallbladder.

Indication: Asthma and diseases of the Liver and Gallbladder.

4) Internal Genitals (MA—TF) (former name: Uterus, Seminal Palace)

Location: In the anterior 1/3 of the triangular fossa.

Functions: Replenishing the Kidney and nourishing Essence, regulating menstruation and astringing leukorrhea, and relieving inflammation and pain.

Indications: Irregular menstruation, dysmenorrhea, leukorrhagia, dysfunctional uterine bleeding, nocturnal emission, prospermia, prostatitis, and hypogonadia.

5) Superior Triangular Fossa (MA—TF) (former name: Lowering Blood Pressure Point)

Location: Anterior and superior of the triangular fossa.

Functions: Lowering blood pressure.

Indications: Hypertension.

5. The tragus points (Fig. 3—6)

1) External Ear (MA—T)

Location: Anterior to the supratragal notch, near the helix.

Functions: Relieving inflammation and pain.

Indications: Inflammation of the external auditory canal, otitis media, and tinnitus.

2) External Nose (MA—T1)

Location: At the point anterior to the center of the lateral aspect of tragus.

Functions: Clearing away Heat and Toxic Materials and relieving inflammation and pain.

Indications: Nasal vestibulitis, rhinitis, and rosacea.

3) Apex of Tragus (MA—T2)

Location: At the tip of the upper protuberance on the border of the tragus.

Functions: Subduing fever and relieving pain.

Indications: Fever and toothache.

4) Adrenal Gland (MA—T)

Location: At the tip of the lower protuberance on the border of the tragus.

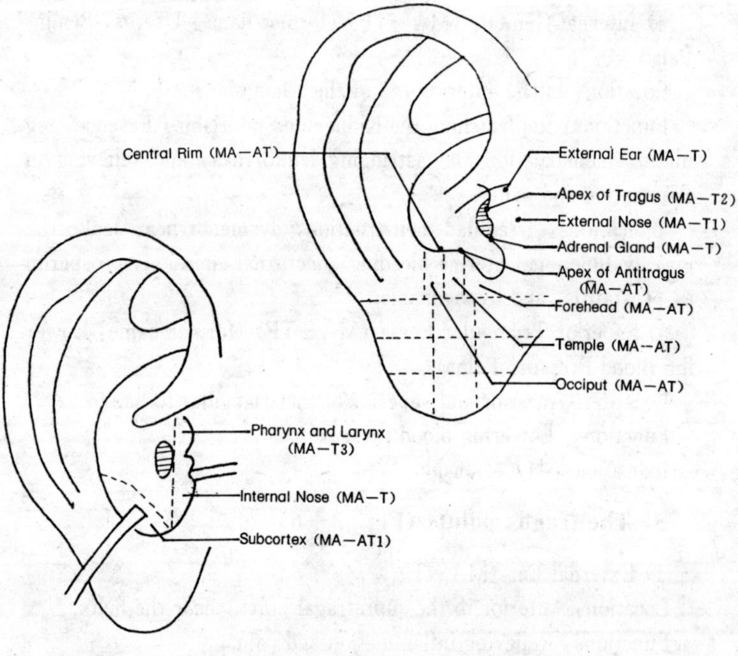

Fig. 3—6 The tragus and antitragus points

Functions: Regulating the secretion of the adrenaline, relieving cough and asthma, clearing away Heat and Dampness, alleviating spasm and pain, expelling Wind, and arresting itching.

Indications: Hypotension, rheumatic arthritis, parotitis, tertian malaria, streptomycin toxic dizziness, asthma, and allergic diseases such as transfusion reaction.

5) Pharynx and Larynx (MA—T3)

Location: At the upper 1/2 portion of the medial aspect of tragus.

Functions: Clearing away Heat and Toxic Materials and relieving sore throat.

Indications: Hoarseness, pharyngitis, and tonsillitis.

6) Internal Nose (MA—T)

Location: At the lower 1/2 portion of the medial aspect of tragus.

Functions: Clearing away Heat and Toxic Materials and clearing the nasal passage.

Indications: Rhinitis, paranasal sinusitis, epistaxis, and nasal obstruction due to Cold.

6. The antitragus points (Fig. 3—6)

1) Apex of Antitragus (MA — AT) (former name: Subduing Asthma, Parotid Gland)

Location: At the tip of the antitragus.

Functions: Relieving cough and asthma, subduing inflammation, and ceasing pain.

Indications: Asthma, mumps, cutaneous pruritus, and epididymitis.

2) Central Rim (MA—AT) (former name: Brain Point, Brain Stem)

Location: At the midpoint between the antitragal apex and antihelix- antitragal notch.

Functions: Replenishing the Spleen and the Kidney, nourishing brain, and tranquilizing the mind.

Indications: Enuresis, auditory vertigo, amnesia, and irregular menstruation.

3) Occiput (MA—AT) (former name: Dizziness Point)

Location: At the posterior superior corner of the lateral aspect of the antitragus.

Functions: Clearing away Heat and checking Wind, tranquilizing the mind and calming the Heart, and nourishing the Liver and improving vision.

Indications: Dizziness, vertigo, headache, insomnia, asthma, epilepsy, myopia, presbytia, car sickness, and sea sickness.

4) Temple (MA—AT) (former name: Taiyang)

Location: At the midpoint of the lateral aspect of the antitragus.

Functions: Tranquilizing the mind and relieving pain, clearing away Heat from the Liver, and promoting vision.

Indications: Migraine, tinnitus, and ametropia.

5) Forehead (MA—AT)

Location: At the anterior-inferior corner of the lateral aspect of the antitragus.

Functions: Tonifying the brain and calming the mind, and dredging Collaterals and relieving pain.

Indications: Headache, dizziness, insomnia, and dream-disturbed sleep.

6) Subcortex (MA—AT1)

Location: On the medial aspect of the antitragus.

Functions: Tonifying the brain, calming the mind, and relieving inflammation and pain. The point has the efficacy of regulating the excito- inhibitory function of the cerebral cortex.

Indications: Pain syndromes, tertian malaria, neurosism, inflammation, pseudomyopia, neurosism, and dysfunction of the vegetative nerve.

7. The inferior concha points (Fig. 3—7)

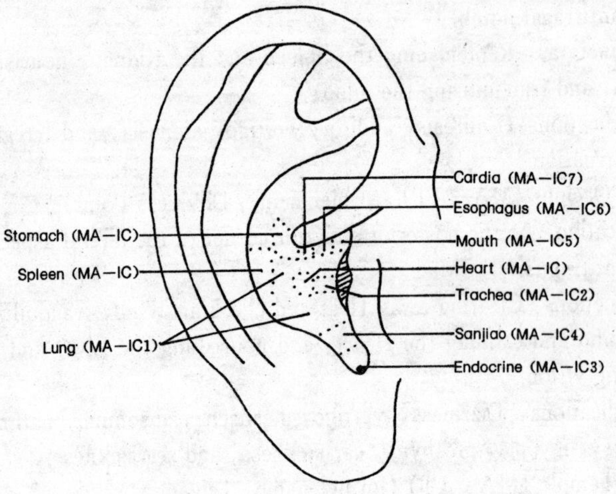

Fig. 3—7 The inferior concha points

1) Heart (MA—IC)

Location: In the central depression of the inferior concha.

Functions: Calming the Heart, tranquilizing the mind, regulating Blood, and eliminating excess Heart Fire.

Indications: Tachycardia, arrhythmia, angina pectoris, acrotism, neurasthenia, stomatitis, and ulceration of the mouth and tongue.

2) Lung (MA—IC1)

Location: Around the central depression of the inferior concha.

Functions: Dispersing the Lung Qi and relieving cough and asthma, dispelling Wind, activating Blood, and arresting itching.

Indications: Cough, asthma, chest stuffiness, hoarseness, laryngitis, acne, flat wart, urticaria, skin pruritus, constipation, withdrawal syndrome, and rhinitis.

3) Trachea (MA—IC2)

Location: Between the orifice of the external auditory meatus and Heart (MA—IC).

Functions: Relieving cough and asthma, removing Heat, and clearing throat.

Indications: Cough, asthma, and acute or chronic pharyngitis.

4) Spleen (MA—IC)

Location: At the posterior and superior aspect of the inferior concha.

Functions: Strengthening the Spleen and the Stomach, invigorating Qi in the Middle Jiao and regulating menstruation.

Indications: Abdominal distention, diarrhea, anorexia, dysfunctional uterine bleeding, leukorrhagia, and auditory vertigo.

5) Endocrine (MA—IC3)

Location: At the base of the inferior concha, interior to the intertragal notch.

Functions: Regulating Qi and menstruation, activating Blood and dredging Collaterals, dispelling Wind and eliminating Dampness, and clearing away Heat and relieving inflammation. The point has the efficacy of regulating the endocrine system.

Indications: Dysmenorrhea, irregular menstruation, climacteric syndrome, acne, diabetes, rheumatic arthritis, malaria, hyperthyroidism, obesity, endocrine dysfunction, and various kinds of inflammation.

6) Sanjiao (MA—IC4)

Location: At the base of the inferior concha, superior to Endocrine (MA—IC3).

Functions: Regulating Intestine and clearing the water passage.

Indications: Constipation, abdominal distention, edema, diabetes, and pain of the lateral aspect of upper limb.

7) Mouth (MA—IC5)

Location: At the anterior 1/3 portion of the inferior aspect of the helix crus.

Functions: Dispelling Wind and dredging Collaterals, clearing away Heat and removing Toxic Materials, and regulating one's taste.

Indications: Facial paralysis, stomatitis, cholecystitis, cholelithiasis and withdrawal syndrome.

8) Esophagus (MA—IC6)

Location: At the middle 2/3 portion of the inferior aspect of the helix crus.

Functions: Regulating the flow of Qi to ease chest oppression and relieve inflammation and spasm.

Indications: Esophagitis, esophageal spasm and dyspnea.

9) Cardia (MA—IC7)

Location: At the lateral 1/3 portion of the inferior aspect of the helix crus.

Functions: Relieving spasm and regulating the Stomach to arrest vomiting.

Indications: Cardiospasm and nervous vomiting.

10) Stomach (MA—IC)

Location: Around the area where the helix terminates.

Functions: Strengthening the Spleen and the Stomach, relieving spasm and stopping pain.

Indications: Gastrospasm, gastritis. gastric ulcer, indigestion, dysfunction of gastrointestine, insomnia and toothache.

8. The superior concha points (Fig. 3—8)

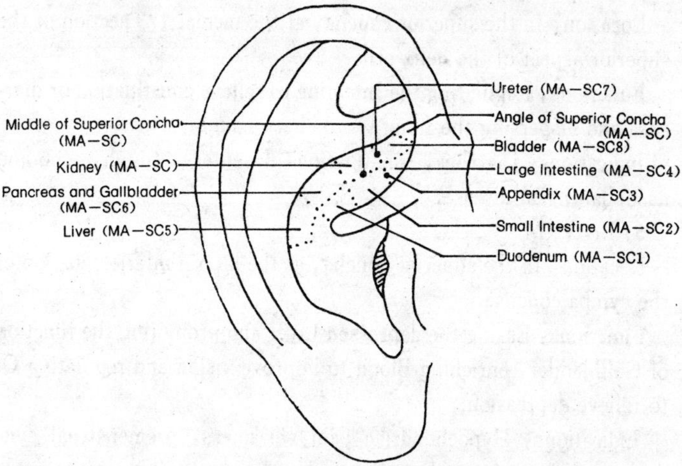

Fig. 3—8 The superior concha points

1) Duodenum (MA—SC1)

Location: In the superior concha, posterior and superior to helix crus.

Functions: Relieving spasm and stopping pain, clearing away Heat and removing Toxic Materials.

Indications: Duodenal ulcer, pylorospasm and cholecystitis, cholelithiasis.

2) Small Intestine (MA—SC2)

Location: In the superior concha, at the superior and middle aspect of helix crus.

Functions: Regulating the Intestine and promoting digestion, calming the Heart and tranquilizing the mind.

Indications: Indigestion, abdominal pain or distension, diarrhea, gastrointestinal dysfunction, tachycardia and arrhythmia.

3) Appendix (MA—SC3)

Location: In the superior concha, between Small Intestine (MA—SC2) and Large Intestine (MA—SC4).

Functions: Relieving inflammation and ceasing pain.

Indications: Simple appendicitis and diarrhea.

4) Large Intestine (MA—SC4)

Location: In the superior concha, at the medial 1/3 section of the superior aspect of the helix crus.

Functions: Regulating the Intestiné to relieve constipation or diarrhea and dispersing the Lung Qi to check cough.

Indications: Diarrhea, constipation, dysentery, cough, acne and nasopharyngeal disease.

5) Liver (MA—SC5)

Location: In the superior concha, at the lateral inferior portion of the cymba conchae.

Functions: Easing the depressed Liver and promoting the function of Gallbladder, enriching Blood to improve vision and regulating Qi to relieve depression.

Indications: Hypochondriac pain, dizziness, premenstrual syndrome, climacteric syndrome, hypertension, pseudomyopia, simple glaucoma, cholecystitis, cholelithiasis, acute conjunctivitis and neurosism.

6) Pancreas and Gallbladder (MA—SC6)

Location: In the superior concha, between Liver (MA—SC5) and Kidney(MA—SC).

Functions: Easing the depressed Liver and promoting the function of Gallbladder, clearing away Heat and removing Toxic Materials, dredging Collaterals and relieving pain.

Indications: Cholecystitis, cholelithiasis, biliary ascariasis, migraine, herpes zoster, otitis media, tinnitus, poor hearing, acute pancreasitis and diabetes mellitus.

7) Kidney (MA—SC)

Location: In the superior concha, inferior to the bifurcating point between superior antihelix crus and inferior antihelix crus.

Functions: Tonifying the Kidney and enriching Essence, clearing and regulating water passage and improving vision and hearing.

Indications: Lumbago, tinnitus, neurosism, pyelonephritis, asthma, enuresis, irregular menstruation, spermatorrhea, prospermia and diarrhea resulting from Kidney deficiency.

8) Ureter (MA－SC7)

Location: In the superior concha between Kidney (MA－SC) and Bladder (MA－SC8).

Functions: Clearing away Heat-Dampness from the Lower Jiao, relieving spasm and stopping pain.

Indication: Colic pain due to ureter calculus, urinary tract infection.

9) Bladder (MA－SC8)

Location: In the superior concha, between Kidney (MA－SC) and Angle of the Superior Concha (MA－SC).

Functions: Clearing away Heat-Dampness from the Lower Jiao and dredging Channels and Collaterals.

Indications: Cystitis, enuresis, retention of urine, lower back pain, sciatica, occipital pain and urinary calculi.

10) Angle of Superior Concha (MA－SC)

Location: At the medial superior angle of the superior concha.

Functions: Clearing away Heat and eliminating Dampness, replenishing the Kidney and enriching Essence.

Indications: Prostatitis, prostatic hyperplasia, urethritis and sexual disorder.

11) Middle of Superior Concha (MA－SC)

Location: In the center of superior concha.

Functions: Clearing away Heat and relieving pain, regulating the Middle Jiao and replenishing the Spleen.

Indications: Abdominal pain and distension, biliary ascariasis andparotitis.

9. The ear lobe points (Fig. 3－9)

1) Eye 1 (MA－L)

Location: On the anterior and inferior side of the intertragal notch.

Functions: Enriching Essence and improving vision.

Indications: Pseudomyopia.

2) Eye 2 (MA－L)

Location: On the posterior and inferior aspect of the intertragal notch.

Functions: Enriching Essence and improving vision.

Indications: Pseudomyopia.

3) Tooth (MA−L)

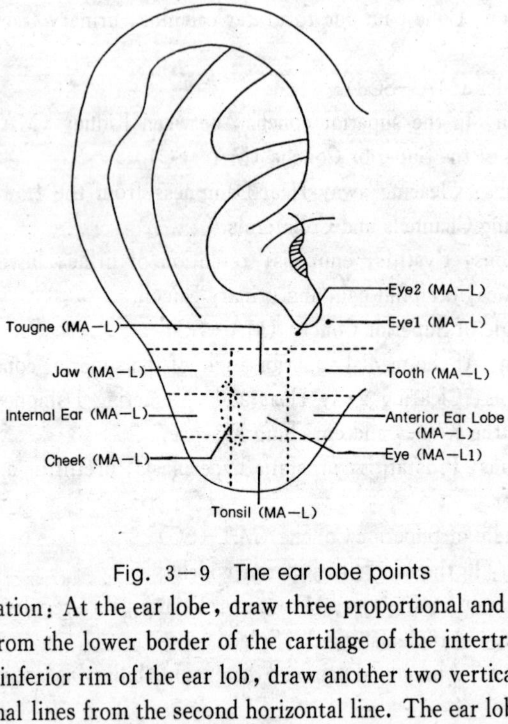

Fig. 3−9 The ear lobe points

Location: At the ear lobe, draw three proportional and horizontal lines from the lower border of the cartilage of the intertragal notch to the inferior rim of the ear lob, draw another two vertical and proportional lines from the second horizontal line. The ear lobe is divided into 9 areas from inward to outward, and upward to downward. The area 1 is Tooth (MA−L); area 2, Tongue; area 3, Jaw (MA−L); area 4, Anterior Ear Lobe (MA−L); around the junction between area 5 and area 6, Cheek (MA−L); and area 8, Tonsil (MA−L). The area 7 and area 9 are empty area without auricular points.

Functions: Relieving inflammation and stopping pain, invigoratingQi and enriching Blood.

Indications: Toothache, periodontitis and hypotension.

4) Tongue (MA-L)

Location: In the second area.

Functions: Relieving inflammation and stopping pain.

Indications: Glossitis and stomatitis.

5) Jaw (MA-L)

Location: In the third area.

Functions: Relieving inflammation and stopping pain and dredging Channels and Collaterals.

Indications: Toothache and dysfunction of tempomandibular joint.

6) Anterior Ear Lobe (MA-L)

Location: In the fourth area.

Functions: Calming the Heart and tranquilizing the mind, relieving inflammation and stopping pain.

Indications: Neurasthenia and toothache.

7) Eye (MA-L1)

Location: In the fifth area.

Functions: Clearing away Heat and removing Toxic Materials, nourishing the Liver and improving vision.

Indications: Acute conjunctivitis, electric ophthalmia, hordeolum, pseudomyopia.

8) Internal Ear (MA-L)

Location: In the sixth area.

Functions: Replenishing the Liver and the Kidney, enriching Blood and improving hearing.

Indications: Internal auditory vertigo, tinnitus and poor hearing.

9) Cheek (MA-L)

Location: Around the juncture between the fifth area and the sixth area.

Functions: Dispelling Wind and dredging Collaterals, relieving in flammation and stopping pain.

Indications: Facial paralysis, trigeminal neuralgia, acne and flat wart.

10) Tonsil (MA-L)

Location: In the eighth area.

Functions: Clearing away Heat and Toxic Materials and relieving sore throat.

Indications: Tonsillitis and pharyngitis.

10. The posterior surface points (Fig. 3—10)

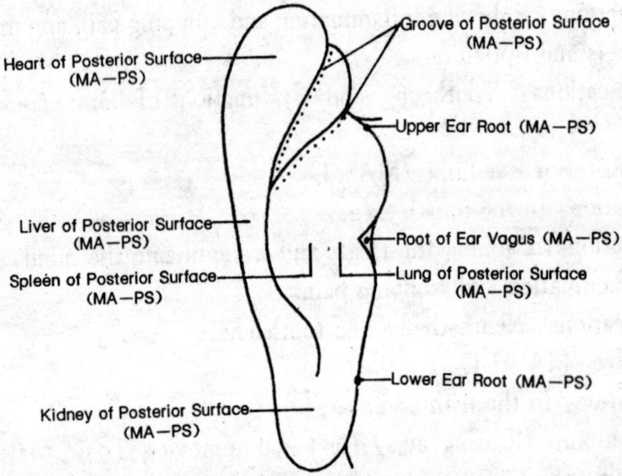

Fig. 3—10 The posterior surface points

1) Upper Ear Root (MA—PS)

Location: At upper most rim of the root of ear.

Functions: Arresting bleeding.

Indications: Epistaxis.

2) Root of Ear Vagus (MA—PS)

Location: Corresponding to the helix crus, at the root of the ear and the junction between the ear back and mastoid process.

Functions: Clearing away Heat and Dampness and relieving spasm and pain.

Indications: Cholecystitis, cholelithiasis, biliary ascariasis, tachycardia, abdominal pain, diarrhea and nasal obstruction.

3) Lower Ear Root (MA—PS)

Location: At lower most rim of the root of ear.

Functions: Invigorating Qi, regulating Blood and tranquilizing the mind.

Indications: Hypotension.

4) Groove of Posterior Surface (MA—PS)

Location: In a "Y" form depression on the back of the ear, which is surrounded by and corresponding to the antihelix, superior antihelix crus and inferior antihelix crus.

Functions: Calming the Liver and sending down the adverse flow of the Liver Qi, dispelling Wind and relieving itching.

Indications: Hypertension and cutaneous pruritus.

5) Heart of the Posterior Surface (MA—PS)

Location: At the upper part of the back of ear.

Functions: Calming the Heart and tranquilizing the mind.

Indications: Palpitation, insomnia and dream-disturbed sleep.

6) Spleen of the Posterior Surface (MA—PS)

Location: At the back region where the helix crus terminates.

Functions: Replenishing the Spleen and Stomach.

Indications: Stomachache, indigestion and anorexia.

7) Liver of the Posterior Surface (MA—PS)

Location: At the region from the Spleen of Posterior Surface (MA—PS) to the place corresponding to the helix.

Functions: Easing the depressed Liver and promoting the function of the Gallbladder, dredging Collaterals and stopping pain.

Indications: Cholecystitis, cholelithiasis and hypochondriac pain.

8) Lung of the Posterior Surface (MA—PS)

Location: At the region from Spleen of the Posterior Surface (MA—PS) to the root of the ear.

Functions: Relieving cough and asthma, dispelling Wind and arresting itching.

Indications: Cough, asthma, and cutaneous pruritis.

9) Kidney of the Posterior Surface (MA—PS)

Location: At the lower part of the back of ear.

Functions: Replenishing the Liver and the Kidney, strengthening bone and enriching Essence.

Indications: Dizziness, headache, tinnitus and neurosism.

Appendix: Empirical Points (Fig. 3—11)

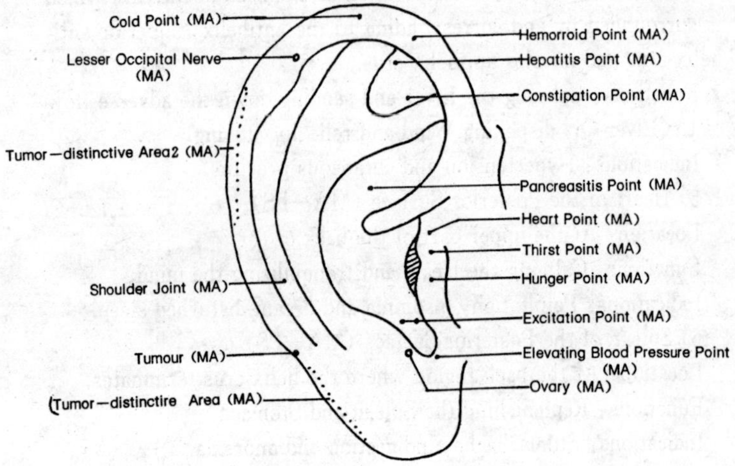

Fig. 3—11 The empirical points

1) Hemorrhoid Point (MA)

Location: At the upper part of the helix, level with the lower border of the superior antihelix crus.

Functions: Clearing away Heat and Toxic Materials, removing Blood stasis and relieving pain.

Indications: Internal hemorrhoid, external hemorrhoid, mixed hemorrhoid and prolapse of rectum.

2) Cold Point (MA)

Location: In the upper part of the helix, slightly anterior to the upper border of the superior antihelix crus.

Functions: Dispersing the Lung Qi to defend the body surface against diseases.

Indications: Prevention and treatment of cold.

3) Tumor-Distinctive Area1 (MA)

Location: In the lower part of the helix, at the upper 2/3 of the line joining Helix 6 (MA—H) with the intersection between helix and the extending line from Stomach (MA—IC) to antihelix-antitragus notch.

Functions and indications: A principal point for diagnosis of malignant tumor.

4) Tumor (MA)

Location: In the lower part of helix, at the mid-point of the upper 1/2 of the line connecting Helix 4 (MA—H) and Helix 5 (MA—H).

Functions and indications: A reference point for diagnosis of malignant tumor.

5) Tumor-Distinctive Area2 (MA)

Location: In the middle part of the helix, at the upper 2/3 of the line connecting Helix1 (MA—H) and Helix3 (MA—H).

Functions and indications: A reference point for diagnosis of malignant tumor, especially digestive tumor.

6) Lesser Occipital Nerve (MA)

Location: In the upper part of the helix, about 0.2 cm interior to the superior border of the helix tubercle.

Functions: Dredging Channels and Collaterals, activating Blood and relieving pain.

Indications: Headache, dizziness, numbness of head and discomfort of neck.

7) Shoulder Joint (MA)

Location: In the scaphoid fossa, at the mid-point between Shoulder (MA—SF4) and Clavicle (MA—SF5).

Functions: Dispelling Wind, activating Blood and dredging Collaterals.

Indications: Periarthritis of shoulder.

8) Constipation Point (MA)

Location: In the triangular fossa, near the lower border of the fossa, superior to Sciatica (MA—AH6) or the middle portion of the inferior antihelix crus.

Functions: Regulating Intestine and relaxing bowels.

Indications: Constipation.

9) Heart Point (MA)

Location: In the depression superior to the apex of tragus, or at the midway between Thirst (MA) and External Ear (MA—T).

Functions: Calming the Heart and mind, and regulating the Heart rate.

Indications: Paroxysmal tachycardia. The point is effective for auricular fibrillation.

10) Thirst Point (MA)

Location: At the midway between External Nose (MA—T1) and Apex of Tragus (MA—T2).

Functions: Nourishing Yin and promoting the production of body fluid to relieve thirst.

Indications: Diabetes mellitus, diabetes insipidus and neurogenic polydipsia.

11) Hunger Point (MA)

Location: At the midway between External Nose (MA—T1) and Adrenal Gland (MA—AT).

Functions: Regulating endocrine and reducing appetite.

Indications: Obesity and hyperthyroidism.

12) Elevating Blood Pressure Point (MA)

Location: In the front of the ear lobe, inferior to the intertragal notch.

Functions: Invigorating Qi and elevating Blood pressure.

Indications: Hypotension.

13) Excitation Point (MA)

Location: At the inferior aspect of antitragus, the lower portion of the line connecting the apex of antitragus with the bottom of antitragus, near Lung (MA—IC1).

Functions: Inducing excitation of the cerebral cortex.

Indications: Lethargy, nocturia, obesity and hypogonadia.

14) Hepatitis Point (MA)

Location: In the triangular fossa, at the junction of the middle and the upper 1/3 of the line connecting Pelvis (MA—TF) and Superior Triangular Fossa (MA—TF).

Functions: Soothing the Liver and promoting the function of Gallbladder.

Indications: Diseases of the Liver and the Gallbladder.

15) Pancreasitis Point (MA)

Location: In the interior angle of superior concha, at the midway between Pancreas and Gallbladder (MA—SC6) and Duodenum (MA—SC1).

Functions: Soothing the Liver and promoting the function of the Gallbladder, relieving inflammation and stopping pain.

Indications: Pancreasitis and diabetes mellitus.

16) Ovary (MA)

Location: In the interior aspect of antitragus, the medial side of the line from the apex to the bottom of antitragus, near Endocrine (MA—IC3).

Functions: Regulating menstruation and enriching Blood, tonifying the Kidney and replenishing Essence.

Indications: Irregular menstruation and hypogonadia.

Ⅳ. Functional Classification of Auricular Points

For the sake of memory and accurate selection of points, auricular points are summarized based on their functions.

1. Calming the Heart and tranquilizing the mind

Heart (MA—IC), Shenmen (MA—TF1), Sympathetic (MA—AH7), Subcortex (MA—AT1), Anterior Ear lobe (MA—L), Occiput (MA—AT), Central Rim (MA—AT), Small Intestine (MA—SC2), Liver (MA—SC5), Kidney (MA—SC), Spleen (MA—IC), Stomach (MA—IC), Heart Point (MA) and Middle Ear (MA—H1).

2. Activating Blood, dredging Collaterals and relieving pain

Finger (MA—SF1), Wrist (MA—SF2), Elbow (MA—SF3), Shoulder (MA—SF4), Clavicle (MA—SF5), Shoulder Joint (MA), Toe (MA—AH), Heel (MA—AH1), Ankle (MA—AH2), Knee

(MA－AH3), Hip (MA－AH4), Buttocks (MA－AH5), Sciatic Nerve(MA－AH6), Neck (MA－AH10), Chest (MA－AH11), Thoracic Vertebrae (MA－AH8), Lumbosacral Vertebrae (MA－AH), Tooth (MA－L), Forehead (MA－AT), Temple(MA－AT), Occiput (MA－AT), Shenmen (MA－TF1) and Subcortex (MA－AT1).

3. Dispelling Wind and relieving itching

Lung (MA－IC1), Shenmen (MA－TF1), Wind Stream (MA－SF), Adrenal Gland (MA－AT), Endocrine (MA－IC3), Subcortex (MA－AT1), Occiput (MA－AT), Ear Apex (MA－H6), Apex of Antitragus (MA－AT) and Points corresponding to the diseased part.

4. Relieving cough and asthma

Lung (MA－IC1), Trachea (MA－IC2), Apex of Antitragus (MA－AT), Shenmen (MA－TF1), Adrenal Gland (MA－T), Endocrine (MA－IC3), Subcortex (MA－AT1), Kidney (MA－SC), Mouth (MA－IC5) and Large Intestine (MA－SC4).

5. Clearing the nasal passage

Internal Nose (MA－T), External Nose (MA－T1), Lung (MA－IC1), Adrenal Gland MA－AT), Wind Stream (MA－SF) and Foreheard(MA－AT).

6. Clearing away Heat to relieve sore throat

Pharynx and Larynx (MA－T3), Mouth (MA－IC5), Lung (MA－IC1), Trachea (MA－IC2), Tonsil (MA－L) and Kidney (MA－SC).

7. Improving hearing

Kidney (MA－SC), Internal Ear (MA－L), External Ear (MA－T), Liver (MA－SC5), Gallbladder (MA－SC6) and Sanjiao (MA－IC4).

8. Clearing away excess Heat from the Liver and improving vision

Liver (MA－SC5), Eye (MA－L1), Eye1 (MA－L), Eye2 (MA－L), Ear Apex(MA－H6), Kidney (MA－SC) and Subcortex (MA－AT1).

9. Soothing the Liver and normalizing the Gallbladder

Liver (MA－SC5), Pancreas and Gallbladder (MA－SC6), Sanjiao (MA－IC4), Sympathetic (MA－AH7), Endocrine (MA－IC3), Liver Yang (MA－H), Middle of the Triangular fossa (MA－TF) and Root of Ear Vagus (MA－PS).

10. Tonifying the Spleen and regulating the Stomach

Spleen (MA－IC), Stomach (MA－IC), Sanjiao (MA－IC4), Large Intes tine (MA－SC4), Small Intestine (MA－SC2), Abdomen (MA－AH), Duodenum (MA－SC1), Sympathetic (MA－AH7), Subcortex (MA－AT1) and Endocrine (MA－IC3).

11. Tonifying the Kidney and nourishing Essence

Kidney (MA－SC), Liver (MA－SC5), Internal Genitals (MA－TF), Pelvis (MA－TF), Endocrine (MA－C3), Sanjiao (MA－SC4), External Genitals (MA－H4) and Central Rim (MA－AT).

12. Calming the Liver to subdue Wind

Liver (MA－SC5), Occiput (MA－AT), Liver Yang (MA－H), Groove of Posterior Surface (MA－PS), Ear Apex (MA－H6), Shenmen (MA－TF1) and Subcortex (MA－AT1).

13. Regulating defecation and urination

Large Intestine (MA－SC4), Small Intestine (MA－SC2), Abdomen (MA－AH), Sanjiao (MA－IC4), Spleen (MA－IC), Kidney (MA－SC), Urethra (MA－H3), Bladder (MA－SC8) and Ureter (MA－SC7).

14. Regulating menstruation and enriching Blood

Endocrine (MA－IC3), Internal Genitals (MA－TF), Liver (MA－SC5), Kidney (MA－SC), Spleen (MA－IC), Central Rim (MA－AT), Sympathetic (MA－AH7) and Shenmen (MA－TF1).

15. Clearing away Heat and Toxic Materials

Ear Apex (MA－H6), Helix 1－6 (MA－H), Liver Yang (MA－H), Tonsil (MA－L), Endocrine (MA－IC3) and Apex of Tragus (MA－AT).

16. Reinforcing Qi to elevate Blood pressure

Elevating Blood Pressure Point (MA), Central Rim (MA－AT), Adrenal Gland (MA－AT) and Heart (MA－IC).

17. Regulating Qi to promote discharge of calculi

Liver (MA－SC5), Pancreas and Gallbladder (MA－SC6), Duodenum (MA－SC1), Large Intestine (MA－SC4), Kidney (MA－SC), Bladder (MA－SC8), Ureter (MA－SC6) and Sympathetic (MA－AH7).

18. **Keeping and promoting beauty**

Lung (MA－IC1), Spleen (MA－IC), Liver (MA－SC5), Kidney (MA－SC), Cheek (MA－L), Central Rim (MA－AT) and Endocrine (MA－IC3).

Clinical Application of Auricular-Point-Pressing Therapy

I. Principles for Selection of Points

The principles for point selection are the theoretical basis for prescription of auricular points in treating diseases. A correct selection of points is the key to the improvement of therapeutic effects. General principles are as follows.

1. According to corresponding area

It is the most commonly used and fundamental principle that auricular points corresponding to the diseased area are selected for treatment, e.g. Stomach (MA—IC) is used for Stomachache, Knee (MA—AH3) for disorders of the knee joint, Temple (MA—AT) for migraine, Forehead (MA—AT) for sinsipital headache, and Lumbosacral Vertebrae (MA—AH) for diseases of the lumbar vertebrae. In addition, positive reaction spots in point locicorresponding to diseased focus are also selected, such as tenderness, deformation, papule and desquamation. For example, for treating periarthritis of the shoulder, apart from Shoulder (MA-SF4) and Clavicle (MA-SF5), positive reaction spots appearing in areas of Shoulder (MA-SF4) and Clavicle (MA-SF5) are also selected. Owing to the different natures and foci of the Stomachache, positive reaction spots may appear in different parts of the point area of Stomach (MA-IC). For instance, reaction spots are frequently found in the area lateral and superior to the end of the helix crus in ulcer of the gastric antrum, and in the medial 1/2 of the line connecting the end of the helix and the interior border of the antihelix. Therefore, selecting these positive reaction spots can improve therapeutic effects. Otherwise, if one always uses the same point to treat stomachache of different natures and foci, the therapeutic results will not be satisfactory. In conclusion, to improve therapeutic efficacy it is necessary to select points corresponding to the disease part as the primary in combination with those vicinal points and/or positive reaction spots .

2. According to syndrome differentiation of Zang-Fu organs and theory of Meridians

1) According to syndrome differentiation of Zang-Fu organs

On the basis of the theory of Zang-Fu organs, points are selected in terms of physiological functions and pathological manifestations of the Zang-Fu organs. Syndrome differentiation of Zang-Fu organs is the characteristic of auricular therapy and the kernel of TCM diagnosis and treatment. The human body is an organic integrated entity having the Five Zang and Six Fu organs as the functional activity center. Since each of the Zang or Fu organs is in charge of physiological functions of certain tissues and organs and they are closely related to each other physiologically, auricular points of Zang or Fu organs relevant to a disease can be selected for therapeutic purpose. For example, select Kidney (MA-SC) for loss of hair because the Kidney has its manifestations in the hair, which is stated in the theory of Zang-Fu organs. Select Lung (MA-IC1) for skin diseases and rhinitis because the Lung controls the skin and has its special opening in the nose. Select Lung (MA-IC1) and Large Intestine

(MA—SC4) for acne because it is considered to be caused by upwards steaming of the stagnant Heat in the Lung and the Stomach and TCM holds that the Lung dominates the skin. Patients suffering from acne mostly have the Yangming Heat syndrome and constipation. Select Heart (MA—IC) for insomnia and dream-disturbed sleep because the Heart takes charge of mental activities. And select Spleen (MA—IC) for profuse menstruation, poor appetite and weakness of four limbs because the Spleen governs circulation of the Blood, transportation and transformation of the food Essence, and the four limbs.

2) According to the theory of Channels and Collaterals

The theory of Channels and Collaterals is the theoretical kernel of acupuncture and auricular-point-pressing therapy as well. For many diseases, points can be selected according to courses of Channels and Collaterals and their exterior-interior relations. For example, Gallbladder (MA—SC5), Stomach (MA—IC) and Bladder (MA—SC8) are selected for migraine, sinsipital headache (pain of the forehead) and occipital headache respectively, because according to syndrome differentiation of Channels and Collaterals, the lateral headache is related to the Gallbladder Channel, the forehead headache related to the Stomach Channel, and the hind headache related to the Bladder Channel. Bladder (MA—SC—8) can also be selected for sciatica when it is manifested mainly in the posterior aspect of the leg because the Bladder Channel runs there. Sanjiao (MA—IC4) is selected to treat pain of the lateral aspect of the upper limb because Sanjiao Channel passes there. Stomach (MA—IC) is selected for toothache of the upper teeth while Large Intestine (MA—SC4) for toothache of the lower teeth because the Stomach Channel enters the upper teeth and the Large Intestine Channel enters the lower teeth. Lung (MA—IC1) is supplemented by Large Intestine (MA—SC4) to treat cough, asthma, and nasal disorders because the Lung and the Large Intestine are exteriorly-interiorly related. Heart (MA—IC) is supplemented by Small Intestine (MA—SC2) to treat ulceration on the oral mucosa and tongue because the Heart has its specific opening in the tongue and it is exteriorly-interiorly related to the

Small Intestine.

3. According to theory of Western medicine

Since many auricular points are located on the basis of Western medicine and named after anatomical terms with their functions conformable to Western medicine, point selection should also be based on Western medicine as well as TCM syndrome differentiation of Zang-Fu organs and Meridians. For example, Adrenal Gland (MA—T) is selected to treat inflammatory diseases, allergic diseases, rheumatism, hypotension and shock because Adrenal Gland (MA—T) can regulate the function of adrenal gland that secretes adrenocortical hormones bringing about antianaphylaxis, anti-inflammation, anti-rheumatism and anti-shock. Sympathetic (MA—AH7) is selected to treat functional disorders of the vegetative nerves because the function of the Sympathetic (MA—AH7) is similar to that of the sympathetic nerve and parasympathetic nerve. Subcortex (MA—AT1) and Sympathetic (MA—AH7) should be selected in the treatment of peptic ulcer because the development of ulcer is associated with the high nervous activities. According to the cortico-visceral interrelationship doctrine, high nervous activities affect the visceral function. Harmful psychic stimulation such as over-fatigue, mental stress and anxiety can cause dysfunction of the cerebral cortex, leading to disorders of the subcortex in regulating secretion, digestion and peristalsis of the stomach. As a result, peptic ulcer develops.

4. According to clinical experience

Auricular therapy is a science both ancient and newly-rising. Medical workers in this field have accumulated certain experiences from clinical practice. Although some experiences have not been acknowledged as theory, they are really effective for certain diseases. Therefore, points can be selected based on these specific experiences. For example, External Genitals (MA—H4) is selected for pain of the lumbus and legs, Ear Apex (MA—H6) and Liver Yang (MA—H) for heptic coma, Occiput (MA—AT) for presbyopia, and Exciting Point (MA) for hypogonadia.

5. According to functions of points

Each auricular point has its respective functions and indications, which should also be taken into account for point prescription. For example, Shenmen (MA—TF1) is a key point for tranquilizing the mind and relieving pain, it therefore is used to treat various painful diseases and neurosism. As a key point for tranquilizing the mind and relieving vertigo, Occiput (MA—AT) is effective for dizziness, drowsiness, car sickness and sea sickness. Wind Stream (MA—SF) has the function of dispelling Wind, arresting itching and antianaphylaxis, thus it is often selected for skin itching, urticaria and other allergic diseases. Ear Apex (MA—H6) and Apex of Tragus (MA—T2) have the function of abating fever, so they are frequently chosen to treat fever.

The above principles for selection of points can be applied separately or jointly. In clinical practice, consideration must be comprehensive, that is, grasping the generality as well as the peculiarity of points, selecting points based on syndrome differentiation as well as clinical experience. In formulating point prescription, select primary points first and supplementary points second to avoid disorder of the point prescription. Definite syndrome differentiation and rational point selection are prerequisite to good therapeutic effects.

Ⅱ. Detection of Auricular Points

Whether or not a point is located accurately affects directly the therapeutic effects of auricular-point-pressing therapy. After definite diagnosis, treatment protocol and point prescription are made, sensitive spot or optimum treatment spot should be detected in the loci of the points selected. The commonly used methods of detection are as follows.

1. Observation

Under the natural light, directly examine the auricle with naked eyes or with the aid of a magnifier to notice if there are positive reactions such as color alteration, deformation, papula, desquamation, etc.

1) Color alteration

The commonly seen are spot-like or patch-like whiteness, redness, grayness, pigmentation, and pallor. Spots of white, yellow or grayish white color circled with redness is also detectable.

2) Deformation

The commonly seen is tubercle or cord-like prominence, second to which is spot-like, patch-like or beading-like prominence.

3) Papule

The commonly seen is spot-like white papula, second to which is a red one. Phlyctenoid or eczematoid patch-like papulae can also be encountered.

4) Desquamation

On the cleaned auricle skin there is an isolated desquamation with definite border. It is the hyaline pure white furfuraceous desquamation like the dandruff falling upon the greasy-coated skin.

2. Pressing

To locate a point more accurately, pressing must be applied on the basis of inspection, which is habitually called Seeing First and Pressing Second. Pressing can be performed with a common probe, specially-made spring probe, or simple tools such as a match stick or a pin. Pressing force should be even and moderate, which, if either too heavy or too light, can affect the accuracy of positiveness. If pain is felt upon pressure, it is considered as positive reaction. There are two commonly-used methods for evaluating pain severity as described below.

1) Positive-negative method

"—" stands for no pain response; "+" for slight pain response; "++" for moderated pain accompanied with slight pain reactions such as winking and frowning; "+++" for severe but bearable pain, accompanied with dodging behavior; and "++++" for severe and unbearable pain.

2) Graduating method Ⅰ° corresponds to bearable pain, Ⅱ° to pain with reactions such as winking and frowning, Ⅲ° to pain with reactions such as shouting out of pain, dodging behavior and refus-

ing to be pressed.

The tenderness of auricular points can reflect to some degree the pathological or functional changes of the diseased organ or part of the body. The appearance or disappearance of these spots and severity of tenderness have a certain relation with the occurrence or recovery, improvement or deterioration of the disease. It can appear along with the onset of a disease and disappear following the recovery. Therefore, tender spots can not only serve as a mark for detecting and locating points, but also provide an evidence for judging the change of the patient's condition. Tender spot may develop in the auricular point corresponding to the diseased organ, in the vicinity of the point, or between two neighboring points.

3. Detection with electric devices

Since electric resistance of the auricular points relevant to a disease is lower than that of the points irrelevant, many electric devices have been developed to diagnose diseases and to ascertain positive reactions. The human body is actually an extremely complicated electrolytic conductor. When a certain tissue or organ is in dysfunction, the abnormal bioelectricity will be reflected on auricular points via Channels and Collaterals and manifested by an obvious drop of electric resistance. These points are high-conductivity spots or sensitive spots.

The auricular point detectors are classified into four types based on different display systems.

1) Acoustics-display type

The signal of the weak direct current passing through the body and auricle is amplified by a transistor amplifier, and then is fed into a loud speaker or earphone to produce sound by which the low-resistance spot is displayed. According to the emerging speed and intensity of the sound and also the change of tone, the positive reaction spot can be analyzed and distinguished from the normal one. This type is the most commonly used in clinical practice.

2) Lamplight-display type

The weak current passing through the body is amplified by an amplifier system and a neon lamp is utilized to emit light by which the sensitive spot is distinguished from the normal one. Because of low resistance and high generating voltage, the auricle skin of the sensitive spot may get burnt, which results in stabbing pain and make it difficult for patients to accept. The other shortcoming is that the lamplight can only show where the diseased part is, but cannot indicate how serious the case is. Therefore, the lightlamp-display type is often used in combination with other types. Besides, it requires looking at the light and the auricular point simultaneously, making it less convenient to manipulate than the acoustics-display type.

3) Meter-display type

It directly measures the electric resistance of each point with a meter displaying indexes by which the sensitive spots can be distinguished from the normal points. Its advantage lies in the capability of showing the electric resistance directly and continuously. Because of the inconvenience due to watching the point and the meter simultaneously, it is more often used in laboratory than in clinical practice.

4) Computer-display type

The positive reaction is displayed by a digital display through data processing and percentage processing. The data can be put into storage banks. Some detectors can directly display the data on the screen, or automatically print out via data recording. Because of the transformation into data, quantification and objectification the computer-display type is more accurate and suitable for scientific research.

Detecting methods are as follows:

1) Line-moving pressing

This is a systematic detection of the whole body, suitable for the general examination of the first-visit patient. It helps to find out pathological changes in each part of the body. Detection is carried out according to the anatomical marks of the auricle, from superior to inferior and from interior to exterior. The general order is as follows: triangle fossa→superior concha→vicinity of the helix crus→inferior concha→ antitragus→intertragal notch-tragus→lobe→antihelix→superior helix crus →inferior helix crus→scaphoid fossa→

helix→posterior surface.

2) Point-moving pressing

This is a purposeful detection often applied for locating points before treatment or for revisit patients. In performing, press with a detecting probe at the area of the point loci or in between two points to search for sensitive spots. When sensitive spots are found, attention should be paid to the loudness of sound and degree of the pain response in order to distinguish the false positive reaction from the true one. The pressure should be even and moderate, neither too heavy nor too light. The time staying in one point should be the same and the speed of detection should be steady and not too fast. Avoid repeated detection on one point.

When the detector of acoustics-display type is applied, judgment is mainly based on the emerging speed and intensity of the sound, and also the change of tone. Meanwhile, the possible tenderness, stabbing pain, deformation, color change, desquamation, papula, etc. should be paid attention to. The electric resistance is divided into three levels as follows:

1) Strongly positive

The sound emerges quickly with a loud tone, often accompanied with stabbing pain. Symbol: "++".

2) Positive

The sound emerges less quickly with lower tone, often accompanied with a feeling of pressing pain. Symbol: "+".

3) Mildly positive

The sound emerges slowly with a weak tone. No feeling of pain presents. Symbol: "±".

The high-conductivity spots detected should be comprehensively analyzed to determine the points for treatment.

The application of electric devices is limited because it needs certain conditions while inspection and pressing methods are more commonly used in clinical practice. The detection is often followed by pressing the point to form a depression, thus facilitating the treatment.

Ⅲ. Classification, Manipulation and Precaution of Auricular-Point-Pressing Therapy

1. Medicinal-seed-pressing therapy

1) Materials

(1) Medicinal seeds: Medicinal seed-pressing therapy is the most commonly-used method at present, for the seeds can be selected according to one's convenience. The following seeds are often selected: *Wang Bu Liu Xing* (Semen Vaccariae), *Lai Fu Zi* (Semen Raphani), *Bai Jie Zi* (Semen Sinapis Albae), *Jue Ming Zi* (Semen Cassiae), *Huang Jing Zi* (Fructus Viticis Negundo) and *Ji Xing Zi* (Semen Impatientis). Small hard pills of Chinese patent medicine, such as *Liu Shen Wan* (Six Miraculous Drugs Pill) and *Hou Zhen Wan* (Relieving Sore Throat Pill) can also be employed. However, Semen Vaccariae is the most widely used because of its smooth and round surface, equal size and hard nature.

Seeds, excluding medicinal pills, are soaked in 75% alcohol or boiling water for several minutes, and then taken out and stored in a glass bottle after being dried in air for later use.

(2) Plate: The plate can be made by yourself. Select a Plexiglas plate of 0.5—0.7 cm thick, process it into a rectangle plate of $14 \times 10\ cm^2$, on which small checks of $0.6 \times 0.6\ cm^2$ are carved out. Each line should be carved no less than 1 mm deep in case the blade goes beyond the line when cutting the adhesive plaster. In the center of each check, drill a hemispherical hollow 0.8 mm in depth and 1.5 mm in diameter. When it is used, put Semen Vaccaria in the hollows, then stick a piece of adhesive plaster (the same size as the plate) on it smoothly and tightly, and then use a blade to cut the adhesive plaster into small checks along the carved line. When performing treatment, the small pieces of plaster, each with a vaccaria

seed, can be taken out with medical forceps or mosquito forceps for use. This kind of plate is available in medical market. If the plate is not available, use a pair of scissors to cut the adhesive plaster into small checks of $0.6 \times 0.6\ cm^2$, stick a seed on the center of each piece, and then put it on the surface of a glass container or a spatula one by one for later use.

2) Manipulation

Sterilize the skin routinely and wait till it is dry, then hold the auricle with the left hand and the forceps or mosquito forceps with the right hand to stick the prepared seed-stuck plaster on the selected points, and then press it tight (Fig. 4—1). The patient is asked to press the seeds 3—4 times per day, 1—2 minutes on each point. The pressure should be limited to the patient's maximal tolerance and subsequently produce sensations of soreness, numbness, distension, pain, etc. Usually, the seeds are left in place for 3—5 days and one ear is treated at a time alternately. Five to ten treatments constitute one therapeutic course.

3) Precautions

(1) For each treatment, the selected points should not be excessive, generally 3—5 and 10 at the most.

(2) During the period of treatment, care should be made to avoid wetting the auricle, which can reduce adhesion and lead to fall of the adhesive tape.

(3) Pressure on the retained seeds should be not too hard and rubbing should be avoided to prevent injury to the skin which may result in infection.

(4) If the patient is allergic to the zinc oxide adhesive tape, please try other auricular therapeutic methods.

(5) It is inappropriate to perform this method when frostbite or inflammation develops on the auricle.

(6) During summer season, the seeds should not be retained too long because of sweating. Two to three days are proper for changing the seeds.

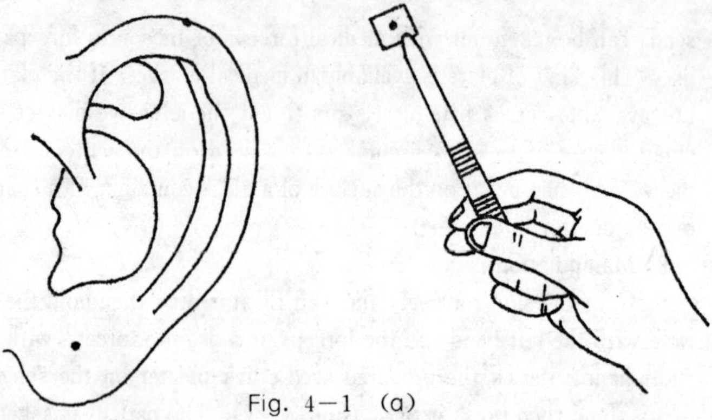

Fig. 4—1 (a)

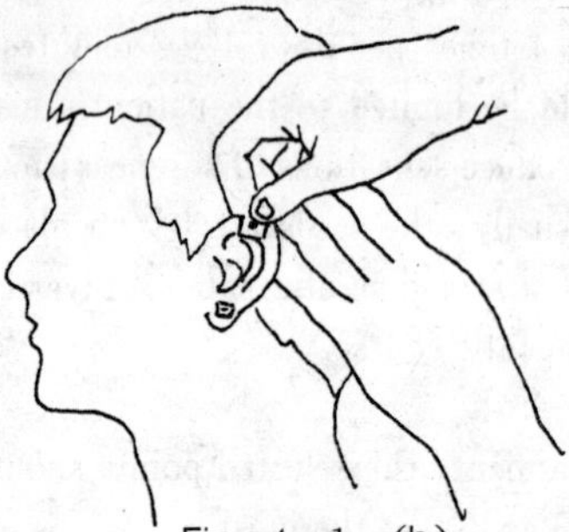

Fig. 4—1 (b)

2. Magnetic-bead-pressing therapy

1) Materials

This is a therapeutic therapy in which the magnetic bead or piece is applied to auricular points to produce therapeutic effects via the magnetic influence on the points. The magnetic intensity of the magnet ranges from 300 GS to 1,500 GS, and the size of magnet should not be large. At present, the specially-made magnetic bead is frequently used.

2) Manipulation

(1) Direct sticking method: Put a magnetic bead or piece in the center of a small piece of adhesive tape and stick it to the selected point. If necessary, stick another one on the opposite aspect of the auricle with their different magnetic polarities opposite to each other, by which the magnetic force can be concentrated to penetrate the

point, thus improving therapeutic effects. In general, no more than four beads are used in each treatment which lasts 3—5 days. After one treatment, stop for 3—5 days and then begin the next. In the Second Municipal Hospital of Beijing, the magnetic bead-pressing therapy was used instead of auricular needling to treat dermatoses such as urticaria, flat wart and neurodermatitis. Analysis of 121 cases revealed that 36% of the patients were cured, 24% were remarkably improved, 33% were mildly improved, and 2% were not improved.

(2) Indirect sticking method: Wrap a magnetic bead with thin absorbent cotton and then put it in the center of a piece of adhesive tape which is to be stuck on to the auricular point. In this way, the side effects of the magnet that directly acts on the skin can be reduced. For instance, when serious perichondritis of the auricle is treated with direct sticking method (two magnetic beads are stuck to a point from the opposite aspect without separation with cotton), local dermonecrosis may be caused due to strong magnetic attraction. For treatment of tinnitus and deafness, magnetic beads that are wrapped with thin cotton can be plugged into the external acoustic meatus. In performing indirect sticking therapy, 2—4 points are proper in one treatment with alternate use of the two ears at intervals of 3 — 4 days. Ten treatments constitute one therapeutic course.

3) Precautions

(1) During the period of treatment, a few patients may develop such adverse reactions as palpitation, dizziness, nausea, fatigue, drowsiness, hot or itch sensation, blister and eccymosis in local area. Mild reactions will disappear spontaneously several minutes or days after starting treatment, while severe reactions will disappear immediately after removing the beads.

(2) In the first treatment, two points are appropriate, no more than four points. Excessive magnetic beads may result in interference among the magnetic fields, thus affecting therapeutic effects.

(3) For some chronic diseases, though the symptoms have disappeared or been improved following treatment, it is necessary to con-

tinue the treatment for a period of time to avoid recurrence.

(4) Discontinue the treatment when any allergic reaction presents.

3. Adhesive-plaster-sticking therapy

1) Materials

This is a therapeutic method in which some kinds of irritant adhesive plasters are stuck to the auricular points. It treats diseases via the drugs contained in the plaster permeating into the points to produce a continuous stimulation.

The commonly-used plasters are as follows: *Xiao Yan Zhi Tong Gao* (Plaster for Relieving Pain and Inflammation), *Xiao Gui Huo Xue Gao* (Plaster for Promoting Blood Circulation with Moschus and Cortex Cinnamomi), *Huo Xue Zhi Tong Gao* (Plaster for Promoting Blood Circulation to Relieve Pain), *Shang Shi Zhi Tong Gao* (Plaster for Dispelling Dampness and Relieving Pain), *Guan Jie Zhi Tong Gao* (Plaster for Relieving Arthralgia). Of the above plasters, *Xiao Yan Zhi Tong Gao* (Plaster for Relieving Pain and Inflammation) is most commonly used because it has a rich source and does not contain moschus.

2) Manipulation

Firstly, clean the auricle or swab it with alcohol cotton ball so that the plaster can be stuck tightly and drugs absorbed well. Then stick the prepared plaster pieces of $0.6 \times 0.6\ cm^2$ on the selected points tightly. The two ears are used alternately with one treatment lasting for 1—3 days, and ten treatments constitute one therapeutic course.

3) Precautions

(1) Some kinds of plasters, such as *Xiao Gui Huo Xue Gao* (Plaster for Promoting Blood Circulation with Moschus and Cortex and Cinnamomi), *Huo Xue Zhi Tong Gao* (Plaster for Promoting Blood Circulation to Relieve Pain) and *Shang Shi Zhi Tong Gao* (Plaster for Dispelling Dampness and Relieving Arthritis), should be used cautiously or prohibitively for pregnant women because of their strong fragrance and high permeability which are helpful for

dredging Channels and Collaterals, promoting Blood circulation to relieve pain, and increasing stimulation.

(2) The plaster should be fresh, and it can be stored in an airtight container. However, a long-stored plaster is not suitable for use.

(3) Plaster-sticking therapy is contraindicated if the auricular skin is wounded.

4. Finger-pressing therapy

This therapy is carried out by pressing the selected points or positive reaction spots with fingers only. It is mostly adopted in case of not having any pressing materials or in emergency. For example, finger-pressing at Stomach (MA－IC) can relieve stomachache, at Ear Center (MA－H1) can cease mild hiccup. In recent years, finger-pressing has been reported to be effective for soft tissue injury.

1) Manipulation

Locate the selected points or positive reaction spots, then place the tip of the thumb on the anterior surface of the auricle and that of the points or positive reaction spots, then plindex finger on the posterior surface opposite to it, or vice versa. Whirling at 30°－60°, slightly press the points for several times, then forcefully for another several times. The force should be concentrated on the point as far as possible.

Since insufficient stimulation will reduce therapeutic effects, pressing force should be strong enough to produce a certain amount of stimulation without injury to the auricular skin. The two ears are used alternately. Each point is pressed for 1－2 minutes or until symptoms are relieved.

2) Precautions

This therapy is contraindicated if the auricle skin is wounded.

Ⅳ. Manipulation of Auricular Pressing

In clinical practice of auricular pressing, attention is paid, just like the body needling and auricular needling, to its manipulation. Different diseases need different manipulations. Generally speaking, mild stimulation is suitable for diseases of the deficiency type and for patients like the elderly, the generally weak, children, and pregnant women; while strong manipulation is suitable for diseases of the excessive type and for young patients with strong constitution. The efficacy of auricular pressing lies in the manipulation skill with finger tips. Though the pressing force is the same, the produced Qi sensation which is an indicator of therapeutic effects may be different with different manipulations such as perpendicular pressing, opposite pressing, oblique pressing and intermittent pressing. Unlike auricular needling, auricular pressing requires the patient to press the points by himself 5－6 times daily. Therefore, the practitioner should introduce the pressing technique in detail to his clients and help them understand and master it. The commonly-used manipulations are as follows.

1. Opposite pressing

Place the thumb and index finger of a hand respectively on the anterior and posterior surface of the auricle and press the stuck seeds in opposite directions till the patient feels a sensation of heaviness, distension, or pain (Fig. 4－2). In case of the patients with high pain threshold, move the two fingers right and left while pressing. Once a pain or distending sensation is felt, stop to press this point continuously for 20－30 seconds. Besides, stick another seed on the other surface of the auricle opposite to the former seed, and then press the two seeds against each other, which can result in a stronger sensation. Pressing is performed on points one by one 3－4 times daily. As an intensive stimulating approach that produces a strong distending pain, it is suitable for the excess syndrome in young people with strong constitution. This pressing method can not only relieve the spasmodic pain of the internal organs but also relieve various somatic pains and acute inflammation.

2. Perpendicular pressing

Place the tip of the index finger perpendicularly on the stuck point and press it till the patient feels a distending pain sensation (Fig. 4—3). At each point pressing lasts for 20—30 seconds and it is repeated 4—6 times at an interval of several seconds. Points are pressed one by one 3—5 times daily. This pressing method produces a weaker stimulation than the opposite pressing method but still a strong stimulating manipulation. It is suitable for the excess syndrome in young people with strong constitution. In addition, it is often applied to those points that are located in the superior concha and inferior concha where the opposite pressing is difficult to perform but strong stimulation is necessary, such as Sympathetic (MA—AH7), Angle of Superior Concha (MA—SC), Ear Center (MA—H1) and Internal Genitals (MA—TF).

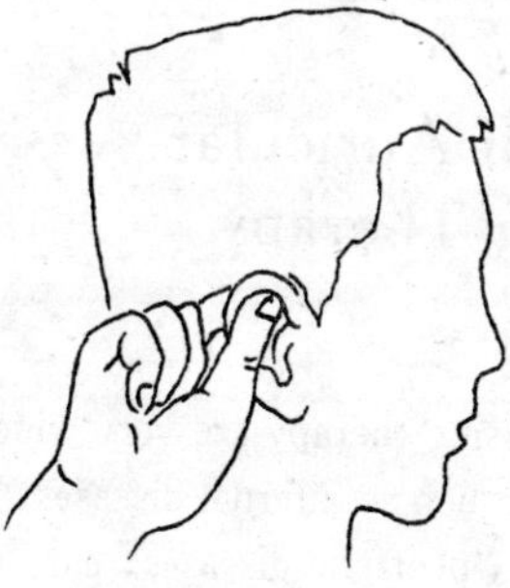

Fig. 4—2

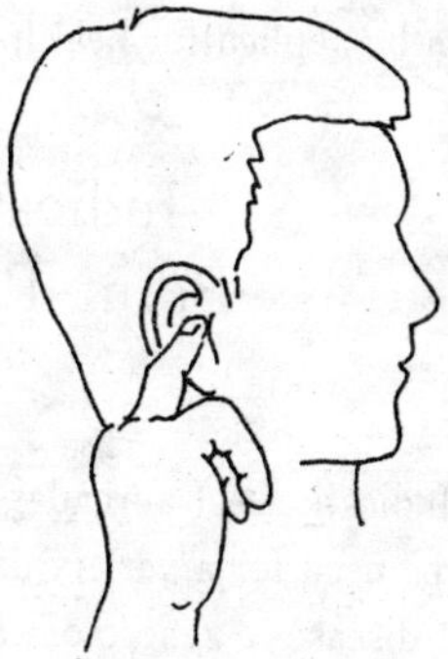

Fig. 4—3

3. Intermittent pressing

Intermittently press the stuck point at intervals of half a second with 20—30 times of press for each point till the patient feels a slight distending pain sensation. This procedure is repeated 3—5 times daily. The pressing force suitable for this method is that able to induce a distending and heavy sensation without severe pain; forceful pressing is inappropriate. As a weak stimulating method, it is suitable for a variety of deficiency syndrome and chronic and functional diseases.

4. Massaging

With the thumb or index finger abdomen, press the stuck point firmly (avoid wounding the skin), then move the finger abdomen clockwise to drive the skin of the point to move till the patient feels a sensation of distension, soreness, or slight stabbing pain. Generally, massaging lasts 3—5 minutes for each point 3—5 times daily. This method elicits a mild stimulation to the point, so it is suitable for those patients with weak constitution due to long duration of illness, and for those who are aged, pregnant, infantile and sensitive to auricular treatment.

Constant massage at certain auricular points is helpful to improve the body metabolism and strengthen the immunological function, resulting in the efficacy of treating and preventing diseases. Therefore it can be applied for health preservation.

V. Indications of Auricular-Point-Pressing Therapy

Indications of auricular-point-pressing therapy are very wide. It can be used for a variety of diseases, such as internal diseases, surgical diseases, gynecological diseases, pediatric diseases, ear, eye, nose and throat diseases, and dermatological diseases. The indications are summarized as follows.

1. Pain syndromes

1) Inflammatory pain

Sore throat, tonsillitis, otitis media, periodinitis, biliary colic due to cholecystitis and cholelithiasis, angitis, etc.

2) Traumatic pain

Sprain, contusion, stab wound, scald, fracture, dislocation, etc.

3) Postoperative pain

A variety of pain following operation, such as pain due to wound or scar.

4) Neurogenic pain

Anginoneurotic headache, migraine, occipital neuralgia, facial neuralgia, trigeminal neuralgia, intercostal neuralgia, sciatica, etc.

5) Tumors pain

Pain resulting from a variety of tumors.

2. Inflammatory diseases

Acute conjunctivitis, keratitis, electric ophthalmitis, tarsadenitis, periodonitis, otitis media, tonsillitis, laryngopharyngitis, acute or chronic trachitis, pleuritis, mastitis, gastroenteritis, appendicitis, pelvic inflammation, orchitis, urocystitis, urethritis, cholecystitis, facial neuritis, etc.

3. Allergic and collagen diseases

Allergic dermatosis, allergic rhinitis, allergic asthma, allergic colonitis, erythema nodosum, rheumatoid arthritis, etc.

4. Neuroendocrine disorders

Neurosism, hysteria, dizziness, hypertension, arrhythmia, gastrointestinal dysfunction, sexual hypofunction, climacteric syndrome, dysmenorrhea, irregular menstruation, amenorrhea, impotence, spermatorrhea, hyperthyroidism, diabetes, obesity, etc.

5. Other chronic diseases

Chronic pain of wrist and leg, cervical spondylopathy, retrograde affection of knee joint, chronic gastrointestinal disorder, sequelae of brain trauma, numbness of limbs, etc.

Treatment of Common Diseases

I. Internal and Pediatric Diseases

1. Cold

Cold, including upper respiratory tract infection and influenza, is the most common exopathic disease caused by bacteria or virus. It may occur around the year but more often in winter and spring. The upper respiratory infection of the nasal cavity, pharynx and larynx, and trachea is manifested mainly by aversion to cold, fever, cough, sore throat and headache. Influenza is characterized by mild symptoms of the upper respiratory tract and obvious systematic manifestations such as chill, high fever and general pain.

In TCM, this disease belongs to the categories of *Gan Mao* (The Common Cold), *Shang Feng* (Attack of Cold) and *Shi Xing Gan Mao* (Influenza). TCM holds that it is caused by invasion of Wind-Cold into the body surface leading to dysfunction of the Lung in dispersing, or invasion of Wind-Heat to the Lung leading to dysfunction of the Lung in purifying and descending.

Point (Fig. 5—1) and method

Main points: Cold Point (MA), Lung (MA－IC1), Internal Nose (MA－T) External Nose (MA－T1), Pharynx and Larynx (MA－T3), Ear Apex (MA－H6), Adrenal Gland (MA－T).

Supplementary Points: Trachea (MA－IC2), Forehead (MA－AT), Occiput (MA－AT), Spleen (MA－IC).

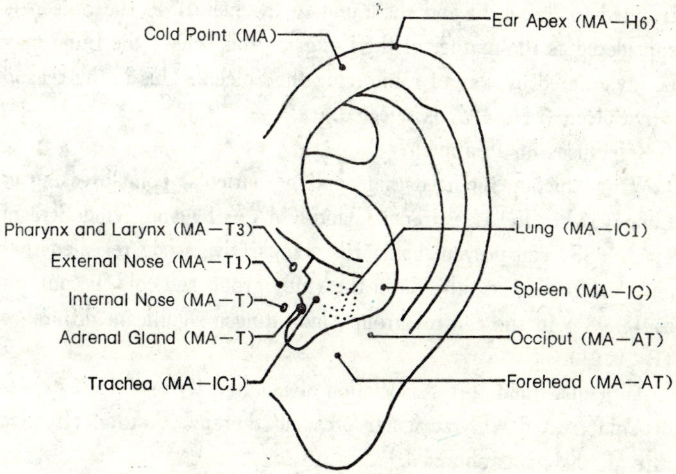

Fig. 5－1 Points for cold

Method: Apply auricular-point-pressing therapy with vaccaria seeds. The opposite pressing or perpendicular pressing is recommended.

Basis for selection of point

Treatment should be based on expelling Wind to relieve external syndrome, removing Heat and dispersing the Lung-Qi. Therefore, Cold Point (MA) is used to expel Wind to relieve Biao Zhen (External Syndrome), supplemented with Lung (MA－IC1) to regulate the Lung-Qi. Internal Nose (MA－T) and External Nose (MA－T1) are used to clear the nasal passage, Pharynx and Larynx (MA－T3) to relieve sore throat, Ear Apex (MA－H6) to clear away Heat, to remove Toxic Materials and subdue fever. Adrenal Gland (MA－T) has the function of anti-inflammation and anti-allergy, which can be strengthened when Lung (MA－IC1) is combined. Add Trachea (MA－IC2) for severe cough, Forehead (MA－AT) and Occiput (MA−AT) for headache, and points corresponding to the diseased area for pain of limbs. In case of persistent high fever, Ear Apex (MA−H6) can be treated with bleeding therapy to improve the function of removing Toxic Materials and clearing away Heat. According to the theory of Five Elements, the Spleen is attributed to the earth and the Lung to the metal, so the Spleen is considered as the mother of the Lung. In this sense, the Lung may be invigorated by way of reinforcing the Spleen. This is the reason why Spleen (MA−IC) is selected.

References for treatment

Wang Zhichun reported that applying auricular-point-pressing at Lung (MA−IC1), Adrenal Gland (MA−T) and Wind Stream (MA−SF) can prevent cold. His comparative study revealed that only 7.67% of the subjects in the study group had cold in contrast to 48.08% in the control group, indicating a significant difference ($P<0.01$).

Auriculoacupuncture Association of Zigong City reported 57 cases of Cold treated with auricular pressing therapy. A total effective rate of 100% was obtained.

2. Bronchitis

Bronchitis is caused by infection of virus and bacteria or stimulation of smoke, dust and chemical substances on the bronchial mucosa. It is classified as the acute and the chronic. Acute bronchitis has a sudden onset, prior to which there are often itching of the throat, unproductive cough, chest pain, fever, headache, and pain of four limbs. One to two days later, the unproductive cough develops into cough with a little sticky or thin sputum, gradually progressing to cough with yellow purulent or white sticky sputum. Chronic bronchitis usually derives from acute bronchitis, manifested by long-term recurrent cough and expectation, possibly accompanied with dyspnea. The cough is aggravated in the morning and at evening and by climatic change, exposure to cold, or catching cold. Acute onset may ensue as a result.

In TCM, bronchitis belongs to the categories of *Ke Sao* (Cough) and *Tan Yin* (Phlegm Retention Syndrome). It is believed to be caused by invasion of the exopathogens taking advantage of Vital Qi deficiency, leading to dysfunction of the Lung in dispersing and descending.

Point (Fig. 5－2) and method

Main points: Lung (MA－IC1), Trachea (MA－IC2), Adrenal Gland (MA－T), Endocrine (MA－IC3), Shenmen (MA－TF1).

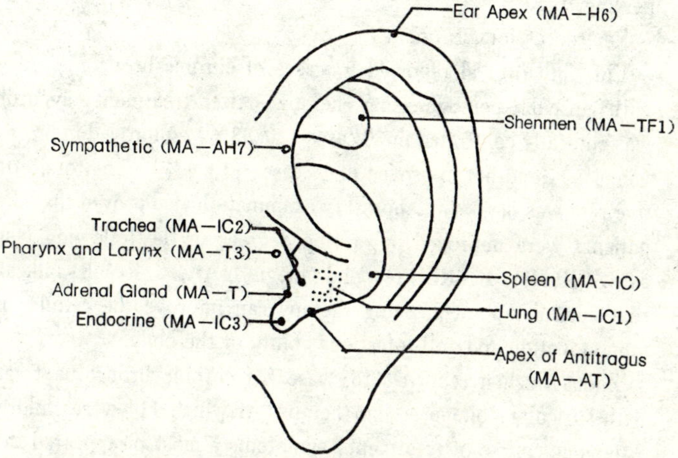

Fig. 5－2 Points for bronchitis

Supplementary points: Apex of Antitragus (MA－AT), Sympathetic (MA－AH7), Ear Apex (MA－H6), Spleen (MA－IC), Pharynx and Larynx (MA－T3).

Method: Apply auricular-point-pressing therapy with vaccaria seeds or magnetic beads. The opposite pressing or perpendicular pressing is recommended.

Basis for selection of point

Lung (MA－IC1) and Trachea (MA－IC2) are selected to regulate the Lung Qi to relieve cough. Having the function of anti-inflammation and antiallergy, Adrenal Gland (MA－T) and Endocrine (MA－IC3) are used to strengthen the body resistance and clear away inflammation. Shenmen (MA－TF1) is combined to tranquilize the mind and relieve cough. Add Apex of Antitragus

(MA−AT), Sympathetic (MA−AH7) for severe asthma, Spleen (MA−IC) to remove Dampness and dissolve Phlegm for profuse phlegm, Pharynx and Larynx (MA−T3) for obvious itching of the throat, Ear Apex (MA−H6) to clear away Heat and Toxic Materials for fever. Since the Lung and the Large Intestine are interiorly-exteriorly related, Large Intestine (MA−SC4) may be added to regulate the flow of Qi and promote the function of the Lung in dispersing.

References for treatment

Liu Xinlian et al reported 97 cases of chronic bronchitis treated with auricular-point-pressing therapy. After treatment, syndrome was clinically controlled in 30 cases (30.93%), improved in 54 cases (55.6%), and not improved in 13 cases (13.4%). The total effective rate was 86.6%. Laboratory examination also proved that these patients were improved in varying degrees in the following tests: skin PHP test, E−RFC test and phlegm IgA test. Results indicated that auricular-point-pressing therapy can improve the cellular immune function and anti-infectious ability of the body.

Zhou Xiuzhen reported 161 cases of chronic bronchitis treated with auricular-point-pressing therapy, of which 114 were children. After one course of treatment, symptoms almost disappeared in 29 cases, were obviously reduced in 130 cases, and were not improved in 2 cases.

3. Bronchial asthma

Bronchial asthma is caused by allergic or anallergic factors leading to hyperactivity of the bronchus. During attacking period, anoxia asthma occurs due to spasm of the bronchial muscle, congestion, edema and increased secretion of the bronchial mucous. The patient manifests himself as chest oppression, short breath, wheezing in the throat and dyspnea. In severe cases, the patient may open the mouth, lift the shoulder and unable to lie flat due to breathlessness. Generally, an episode of attack lasts several minutes. If dyspnea is constant and the patient has a blue complexion, this is called status asthmaticus.

In TCM, bronchial asthma is in the categories of *Xiao Zhen* (Asthma with Wheezing) and *Chuan Zhen* (Asthma). It is believed to be caused by invasion of exopathic Wind-Cold, Wind-Heat, aspiration of dust, smoke, or improper diet, leading to accumulation of pathogens in the Lung and dysfunction of the Lung in dispersing and descending. It may also be resulted from innate deficiency or a prolonged disease leading to failure of the Kidney in receiving Qi.

Point (Fig. 5—3) and method

Main points: Lung (MA—IC1), Trachea (MA—IC2), Adrenal Gland (MA—T), Apex of Antitragus (MA—AT), Endocrine (MA—IC3), Wind Stream (MA—SF), Sympathetic (MA—AH7).

Supplementary points: Shenmen (MA—TF1), Large Intestine (MA—SC4), Kidney (MA—SC), Spleen (MA—IC).

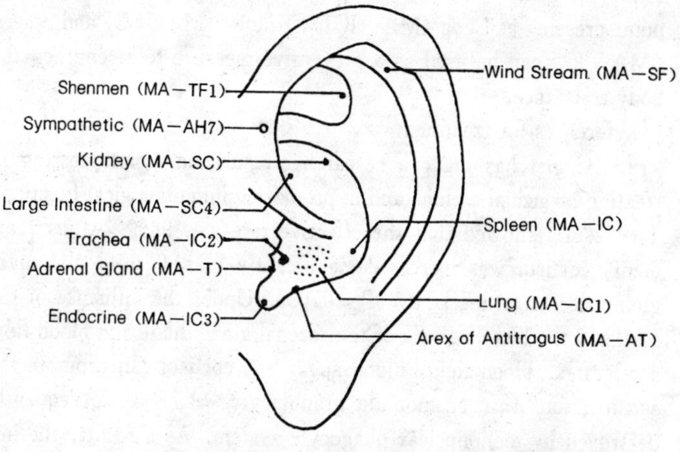

Fig. 5—3 Points for bronchial asthma

Method: Apply auricular-point-pressing therapy with vaccaria seeds or magnetic beads. The opposite pressing or perpendicular pressing is recommended.

Basis for selection of point

Primary therapeutic principle should be dispersing the Lung Qi and relieving asthma. Lung (MA—IC1) and Trachea (MA—IC2) are selected and treated with a rather strong stimulating approach to disperse and regulate the Lung Qi. Apex of Antitragus (MA—AT) is used to relieve cough and asthma. Adrenal Gland (MA—T), Endocrine (MA—IC3) and Wind Stream (MA—SF) are used to desensitize the body and enhance the immunity. Sympathetic (MA—AH7) is used to inhibit vagal excitation and alleviate bronchospasm. Combined use of the above points can smooth the air passage and disperse the Lung Qi to relieve asthma. Large Intestine (MA—SC4), the point interiorly-exterioly related to the Lung (MA—IC1), is used to strengthen the above points in smoothing the Lung Qi. TCM holds that the Lung is the dominator of Qi, while the Kidney is the root of Qi. Deficiency of the Kidney which fails to receive Qi will bring about adverse flow of Qi resulting in asthma. Therefore, for long-term recurrent cases, Kidney (MA—SC) is added to tonify the Kidney in receiving Qi. During convalescence, auricular-point-pressing at Lung (MA—IC1), Kidney (MA—SC) and Spleen (MA—IC) can be used as a preventive measure to strengthen the body resistance.

References for treatment

Li Banglei has made a research on auricular-point-pressing in treating bronchial asthma and in promoting immunological function. The results showed that the effective rate was 96%. After treatment, cortisol was increased significantly ($P<0.001$) and myoglobin decreased markedly ($P<0,05$). Under the influence of the cortisol, the blood vessels of the adrenal gland dilate and blood flow accelerates. blood lipid, blood sugar and cortisol can promote the sensitization of the eosinophilic granulocytes which are subsequently destroyed by mononuclear phagocyte system. As a result, the immunologic function is strengthened.

Zhao Zixian reported 50 cases of asthma with auricular-point-pressing therapy. Symptoms were controlled in 12 cases marked by asthma being controlled for over one month without any need for medicine; basically controlled in 27 cases marked by decreased dosage by 2/3; mildly improved in 10 cases marked by relieved symptoms but medicine was needed to maintain the effects; and failed to respond in 1 case. The total effective rate was 98%.

Hu Jiuheng reported 93 cases of infantile bronchial asthma treated with auricular-point-pressing therapy. Of them, 62 cases were cured (66.7%), 11 were markedly improved (11.8%), 13 were mildly improved (14%), and 7 had no response (7.5%). The total effective rate was 92.5%.

4. Arrhythmia

Arrhythmia is a common symptom, including sinus arrhythmia, tachycardia, various premature beat, bradycardia, auricular fibrillation, etc. It can be caused by cardiac pathological changes or dysfunctional vegetative nerve. The main manifestations are palpitation, shortness of breath, discomfort of the precordial region, dream-disturbed sleep, a tendency to be tightened, and deep thin or knotted intermittent pulse.

In TCM, arrhythmia belongs to the categories of *Jing Ji* (Palpitation) and *Zheng Zhong* (Palpitation with a Distress Feeling). It is believed to be caused by deficiency of Qi and Blood resulting in malnutrition of the Heart.

Point (Fig. 5—4) and method

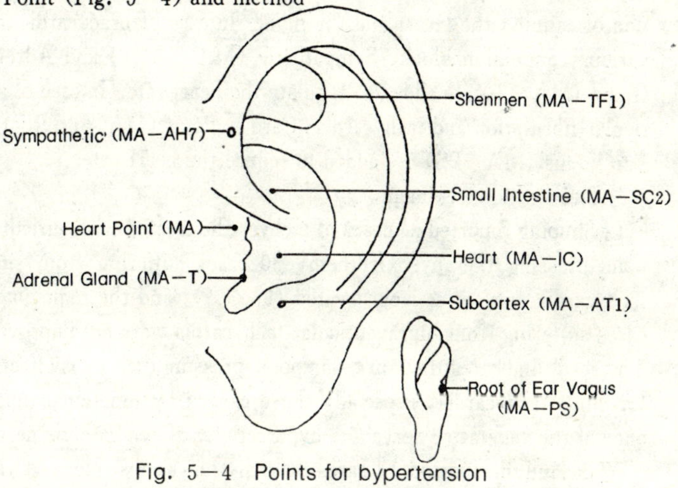

Fig. 5—4 Points for bypertension

Main points: Heart (MA—IC), Small Intestine (MA—SC2), Shenmen (MA—TF1), Subcortex (MA—AT1).

Supplementary points: Sympathetic (MA－AH7), Adrenal Gland (MA－T), Cardiac Point (MA), Root of Ear Vagus (MA－PS).

Method: Apply auricular-point-pressing therapy with vaccaria seeds or magnetic beads. The perpendicular pressing is recommended.

Basis for selection of point

Treatment should be based on the therapeutic principle of nourishing Blood and invigorating Qi, calming the Heart and tranquilizing the mind. The Heart is in charge of Blood and vessels and mental activities. Therefore, Heart (MA－IC) is selected to enrich Blood and activate vessels, to calm the Heart and tranquilize the mind. Modern research has confirmed that stimulating Heart (MA－IC) performs biphasic beneficial regulatory efficacy on Heart rate and improves cardiac function. The Heart and the Small Intestine are interiorly-exteriorly related, so Small Intestine (MA－IC2) is used to reinforce the efficacy of Heart (MA－IC) in regulating the heart rate and strengthening the cardiac function. Shenmen (MA－TF1) and Subcortex (MA－AT1) are used for insomnia, frequent dream and susceptibility to fear and fright, for they have the function of calming the Heart and the mind. In case of bradycardia and various conduction block, Sympathetic (MA－AH7) and Adrenal Gland (MA－T) are added to regulate the heart rate. In case of auricular fibrillation and tachycardia, Cardiac Point (MA) and Root of Ear Vagus (MA－PS) are added to reduce the heart rate.

References for treatment

Li Shuping reported 34 cases of tachycardia treated with auricular-point-pressing therapy. Of them, 30 cases suffering from sinus tachycardia were effectively treated (93.3%), and the remaining 4 cases suffering from supraventicular tachycardia were not improved. The result indicated that auricular-point-pressing therapy is effective for sinus tachycardia, especially those caused by functional imbalance of the vegetative nerve and hyperactivity of sympathetic nerve.

Wan Huilun reported 13 cases of arrhythmia subsequent to viral myocarditis treated with vaccaria seed-pressing therapy. Treatment was carried out every 3－5 days with one course consisting of 10 sessions. Result: all of the patients were cured. Of them, 10 patients recovered within one course, 2 within one and a half courses, and 1 within two courses.

5. Hypertension

Hypertension is characterized by abnormal rising of the arterial pressure, mostly occurring in middle-aged and elderly people. It is classified into two types: the primary and the secondary. The cause of primary hypertension remains uncertain. Generally, dysfunction of the high nervous activity is believed to be related with it. The secondary hypertension, also called symptomatic hypertension, is mostly caused by urinary diseases, intracranial diseases, or endocrine disorders. Primary hypertension manifests itself by headache, distending feeling of the head, dizziness, palpitation, insomnia, blurred vision and numbness of the extremities. Blood pressure is at least 21.3/12.7 kPa (160/95 mmHg).

Clinically, hypertension is divided into three periods:

Period Ⅰ: Blood pressure has reached the level of hypertension, however, no complications of the heart, brain or kidney occur.

Period Ⅱ: Blood pressure has reached the level of hypertension, and at least one of the following abnormalities is founded: ① Left ventricular dilatation detected by physical examination, X-ray, ECG, or ultrasonography; ② General or limited arteriostenosis revealed by examination of the optical fundus; ③ Proteinuria and/or mild increase of the plasma creatinine.

Period Ⅲ: Blood pressure has reached the level of hypertension, and one or more of the following abnormalities is founded: ① Cerebrovascular accident or hypertensive encephalopathy; ② Failure of the left heart; ③ Renal failure; and ④ Retinal hemorrhage or exudation, with or without papilledema.

In TCM, hypertension belongs to the categories of *Tou Tong* (Headache), *Xuan Yun* (Dizziness), *Gan Yang* (Liver Yang Syndrome), etc. It is considered to be caused by hyperactivity of the Liver Yang due to constitutional excess of Yang Qi, or malnutrition of the Liver due to deficiency of the Kidney Yin.

Point (Fig. 5—5) and method

Main points: Groove of Posterior Surface (MA—P), Ear Apex (MA—H6), Heart (MA—IC), Liver (MA—SC5), Kidney (MA—SC), Sympathetic (MA—AH7), Subcortex (MA—AT1)

Supplementary points: Forehead (MA—AT), Temple (MA—AT), Occiput (MA—AT), Shenmen (MA—TF1)

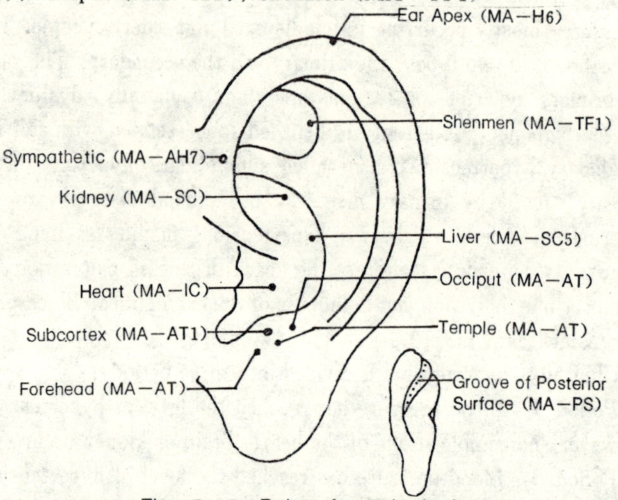

Fig. 5—5 Points for arrhythmia

Method: Mostly apply auricular-point-pressing therapy with vaccaria seeds, magnetic beads, or cassia seeds. The opposite pressing or perpendicular pressing method is recommended.

Basis for selection of point

Treatment should be based on nourishing Yin and suppressing Yang and calming the Liver to cease Wind. Heart (MA—IC) and Kidney (MA—SC) nourish Yin and benefit Blood, and Liver (MA—SC5) calms the Liver, suppresses Yang and subsides the Wind, so they are selected. Groove of Posterior Surface (MA—PS) is an empirical point for treatment of hypertension. Ear Apex (MA—H6) is used to dispel Heat, to refresh the head, to tranquilize the mind and drop blood pressure. Subcortex (MA—AT1) and Sympathetic (MA—AH7) are used to regulate vasomotoricity and relieve vasospasm. For case with severe distending headache, Forehead (MA

—AT) and Temple (MA—AT) are added. For case with severe dizziness, Occiput (MA—AT) is added. For case with insomnia, Shenmen (MA—TF1) is added.

References for treatment severe dizzines

Wang Jinru et al reported 90 cases of hypertension treated with auricular-point-pressing therapy, among which 16 cases were in period I of hypertension and 74 in period Ⅱ. Vaccaria seeds were used for pressing and the seeds were changed every other day with 12 treatment sessions constituting one therapeutic course. Treatment was continued for successive two courses. Criteria for effect evaluation were as follows: Marked improvement: After one course of treatment, blood pressure restored to normal in patients of period I or dropped by 2.66—4 kPa in patients of period Ⅱ; dosage of hypotensor was reduced or withdrawn. Mild improvement: After one course of treatment, headache and dizziness were ameliorated; diastolic pressure dropped by 1.33 kPa or so. No improvement: After one course of treatment, blood pressure remained unchanged. Results: Of the 16 hypertensive cases in period Ⅰ, blood pressure restored to normal; of the 74 hypertensive cases in period Ⅱ, 26 showed marked effect (35.1%), 46 showed mild effect (62.2%), and 2 showed no effect (2.7%). The results suggested that for period I of hypertension, satisfactory efficacy can be obtained with single auricular-point-pressing therapy, while for period Ⅱ of hypertension, oral medicine is needed. Combined use of auricular point pressing therapy and medicine is more effective than single use of medicine.

Yu Peng et al reported 100 cases of primary hypertension treated with auricular-point-pressing with vaccaria seed. Among 26 cases in period Ⅰ, 19 cases were markedly improved, 7 cases were partially improved; 100% of the patients withdrew or reduced their medicine. Among 50 cases in period Ⅱ, 17 cases were markedly improved, 7 cases were partially improved, and 10 cases were not improved; 80% of the patients withdrew or reduced dosage of their medicine. Among 24 cases in period Ⅲ, 2 cases were markedly improved, 12 cases were partially improved, and 10 were not improved; only 58.3% of the patients withdrew or reduced dosage of their medicine.

6. Hypotension

Hypotension refers to that the brachial arterial blood pressure measured with routine method is lower than 12/8 kPa, or 13.33 kPa in people over 65 years old. It can be classified into two categories: the acute and the chronic. The acute type manifests itself by a sudden and obvious drop of blood pressure from a normal or slight abnormal high level, accompanied with two main clinical syndromes of syncope and shock. The chronic type includes constitutional hypotension, orthostatic hypotension, and those resulting from endocrine disorders, chronic exhaustive diseases, malnutrition, or cardiovascular diseases.

In TCM, hypertension belongs to the categories of *Xuan Yun* (Dizziness), and *Xu Lao* (Consumptive Disease). It is considered to be caused by deficiency of Qi and Blood.

Point (Fig. 5-6) and method

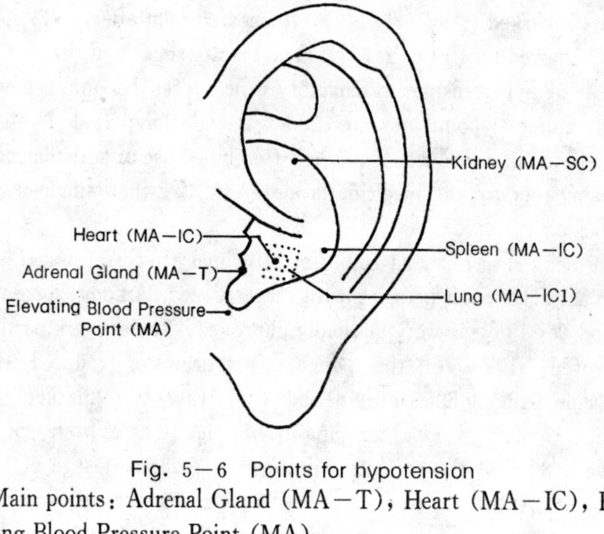

Fig. 5-6 Points for hypotension

Main points: Adrenal Gland (MA-T), Heart (MA-IC), Elevating Blood Pressure Point (MA).

Supplementary points: Kidney (MA—SC), Spleen (MA—IC), Lung (MA—IC1).

Method: Apply auricular-point-pressing therapy with vaccaria seeds. The intermittent pressing is recommended. Finger-pressing is applicable.

Basis for selection of point

Treatment should be based on the therapeutic principle of invigorating Qi and Blood and tonifying the Heart and Vessels. Heart (MA—IC) is selected to promote Blood circulation, to reinforce the Heart, nourish Blood, and to activate pulse. Adrenal Gland (MA—T) has the function of regulating vasomotoricity and elevating blood pressure. Elevating Blood Pressure Point (MA) is an empirical point in raising blood pressure. Kidney (MA—SC) and Spleen (MA—IC) are used to invigorate the Spleen and tonify the Kidney. Lung (MA—IC1) is used to reinforce the Lung Qi to facilitate the Heart in driving the flow of Blood. Combined use of the above points can achieve the effects of enriching Blood, activating pulse, invigorating Qi and raising blood pressure.

References for treatment

Wu Xinfa et al reported that stimulating Heart (MA—IC) produced some influence on cardiac pumping capability of the hemorrhagic shock rabbit. Experimental results revealed that needling Heart (MA—IC) could improve heart failure of the shock rabbit, manifested by elevated SV, increased CO and CL, enlarged dz/dt-P impedance cardioring, and raised blood pressure. As a result, blood perfusion of tissues and organs was ameliorated, which was helpful in preventing microcirculation dysfunction.

Liang Shuzhong et al reported that Adrenal Gland (MA—T) has the function of regulating adrenal gland and adrenocortical hormones. It also performed influence on various cardiac functions via possibly inducing secretion of various adrenocortical hormones. The efficacy of needling Heart (MA—IC) on the cardiac function was of biphasic beneficial regulation, namely, elevating blood pressure in case of hypotension while lowering it in case of hypertension.

7. Coronary heart disease

Coronary heart disease is caused by coronary atherosclerosis leading to myocardial ischemia and hypoxia, manifested mainly by angina pectoris, myocardial infarction, arrhythmia, heart failure and cardiac enlargement. ECG may show myocardial ischemia and loading test presents positive changes correspondingly.

In TCM, angina pectoris and myocardial infarction belong to the categories of *Xiong Bi* (Qi Obstruction of the Chest), *Zhen Xin Tong* (True Stenocardia) and *Jue Xin Tong* (Precordial Pain).

Point (Fig. 5−7) and method

Main points: Heart (MA−IC), Small Intestine (MA−SC2), Subcortex (MA−AT1), Sympathetic (MA−AT7).

Supplementary points: Chest (MA−AH11), Heart Point (MA), Shenmen (MA−TF1).

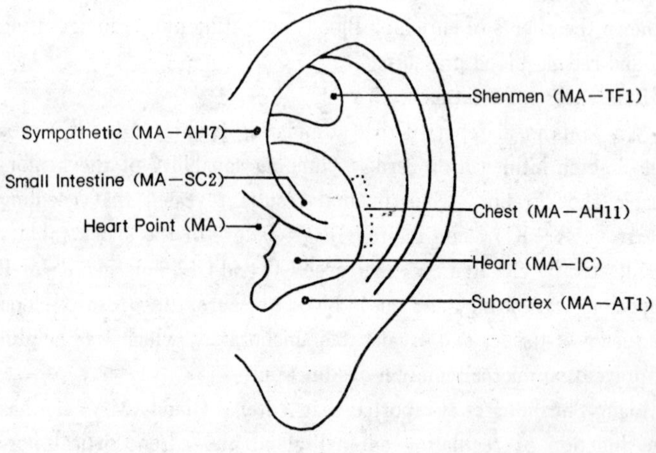

Fig. 5−7 Points for coromary heart disease

Method: Mostly apply auricular-point-pressing therapy. Plaster-sticking therapy is also applicable with the *She Xiang Zhuang Gu Gao* (Plaster for Strengthening the Bone Mainly with Moschus) or *Xiang Gui Hou Xue Gao* (Plaster for Promoting Blood Circulation with Moschus and Cortex Cinnamomi).

Basis for selection of point

As a corresponding point to the diseased part, Heart (MA—IC) is used to improve myocardial ischemia and hypoxia and enhance myocardial function. Since the Small Intestine is exteriorly-interiorly related with the Heart, Small Intestine (MA—SC2) is selected to assist Heart (MA—IC) in ameliorating the cardiac blood circulation and strengthening the myocardial function, subsepuently invigorating Qi, activating Blood flow and removing Blood stasis to relieve pain. Subcortex (MA—AT1) and Sympathetic (MA—AT7) can regulate vasomotoricity and improve coronary blood supply. For cases with fullness or pain of the chest, Chest (MA—AH11) and Shenmen (MA—TF1) are added to regulate the flow of Qi and soothe the chest. For cases with arrhythmia, Heart Point (MA) is added to regulate the Heart rate.

References for treatment

Wang Lei reported 42 cases of myocardial ischemia treated with auricular-point-pressing therapy. Of the 42 cases, 16 cases were cured (40%), 20 cases were remarkably improved (50%), and 4 cases did not respond (10%). The total effective rate was 90%. ECG was improved in all of the markedly effective cases, manifested by basically normalized S—T and T. The author believed that Heart (MA—IC) can regulate the flow of Qi and Blood and improve myocardial blood supply, thus promoting the recovery of the damaged myocardium.

Wei Chijing reported 21 cases of coronary heart disease treated with pressing vaccaria seeds at auricular points. The seeds were changed every 3—5 days with one therapeutic course consisting of 10 treatments. Main points used were Heart (MA—IC) and Small Intestine (MA—SC2). Result: Clinical symptoms disappeared and ECG was normalized in 7 patients after 5 treatments, and in the remaining 14 cases after 10 treatments. The short-term effective rate was 100%.

Wu Xinfa et al reported the experimental effects of puncturing Heart (MA—IC) on cardiac blood circulation, manifested by statistically significant increase of the cardiac pumping function index, heart rate, stroke volume, kinemia and cardiac index according to impedance cardiogram. The results demonstrated that Heart (MA-IC) has the function of strengthening the myocardial contractive power, which provides an experimental basis for clinical practice.

Remarks

Auricular point therapy presents certain effectiveness for coronary heart disease. However, attention should be paid to the changes of EKG. Even when EKG improves or returns to normal, treatment is still needed for a certain period to fortify the efficacy.

8. Acute gastroenteritis

Acute gastroenteritis refers to acute inflammation of gastrointestinal tract due to eating or drinking too much , or food contaminated by bacteria or toxins. It occurs more often in summer and fall and is manifested mainly by abdominal pain, diarrhea and vomiting. Acute gastroenteritis develops suddenly with frequent thin or even watery diarrhea ten or more times daily. Severe vomiting and diarrhea may cause water and electrolyte imbalance.

In TCM, acute gastroenteritis belongs to the categories of *Xie Xie* (Diarrhea) and *Ou Tu* (Vomiting). It is considered to be caused by improper diet or invasion of exthopagens impairing the gastrointestinal tract, thus resulting in dysfunction of Qi activities and conveyance of the gastrointestinal tract.

Point (Fig. 5-8) and method

Main points: Stomach (MA-IC), Spleen (MA-IC), Large Intestine (MA-IC4), Small Intestine (MA-IC2), Sympathetic (MA-AH7).

Supplementary points: Abdomen (MA-AH), Shenmen (MA-TF1), Cardia (MA-IC7).

Method: Mostly apply auricular-point-pressing therapy with vaccaria seeds. The perpendicular pressing method is recommended.

Basis for selection of point

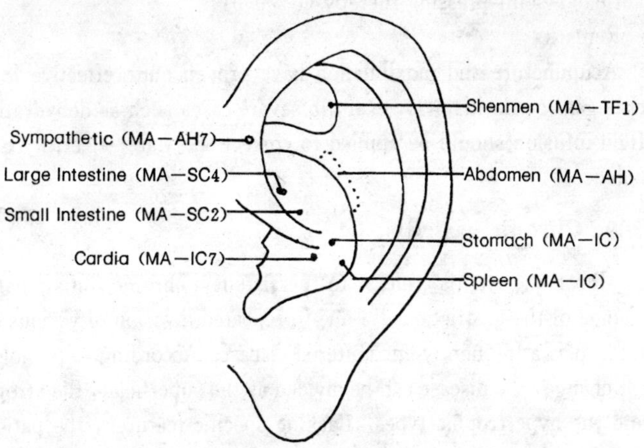

Fig. 5—8 Points for acute gastroenteritis

Primary therapeutic principle should be regulating the gastrointestinal Qi activities. Stomach (MA — IC), Spleen (MA — IC), Large Intestine (MA — IC4) and Small Intestine (MA — IC2) are used to invigorate the Spleen and Stomach, to regulate the transportation and transformation functions of the Stomach and Intestine, consequently relieving vomiting and diarrhea. Sympathetic (MA—AH7) is adopted to relax the spastic visceral smooth muscle to stop pain. For cases with severe diarrhea and abdominal pain, add Abdomen (MA—AH) to regulate bowels and cease diarrhea. For cases with severe vomiting, add Shenmen (MA—TF1) and Cardia (MA—IC7) to tranquilize the mind, to lower the adverse flow of the Stomach Qi to stop nausea and vomiting.

References for treatment

Chi Zhanping et al reported 256 cases of acute gastroenteritis treated with auricular-point-pressing at Spleen (MA — IC) and Large Intestine (MA—SC4) in combination with bloodletting therapy at Ear Apex (MA—H6). All of the patients were cured after only one treatment. In comparison with the control groups treated with oral use of antibiotics and antispasmodics as to the cure rate of one day treatment, there was a significant difference in favor of the auricular-point-pressing therapy ($P<0.01$).

Remarks

Acupuncture and moxibustion have proven quite effective for acute gastroenteritis. However, in severe cases such as dehydration, fluid infusion should be applied to correct the water-electrolyte imbalance.

9. Chronic gastritis

Chronic gastritis refers to persistent, chronic inflammatory change of the gastric mucosa due to repeated invasion of various factors. It is a frequently encountered disease. According to pathological change, the disease can be divided as the superficial, the atrophic and the hypertrophic types. Lacking specific features, the patients suffering from chronic gastritis often complain of distension of the upper abdomen, stomachache, belching, anorexia, acid regurgitation, or discomfort of the stomach when they see a doctor.

In TCM, chronic gastritis belongs to the categories of *Wei Wan Tong* (Stomachache) and *Pi Man* (Fullness of Abdomen).

Point (Fig. 5—9) and method

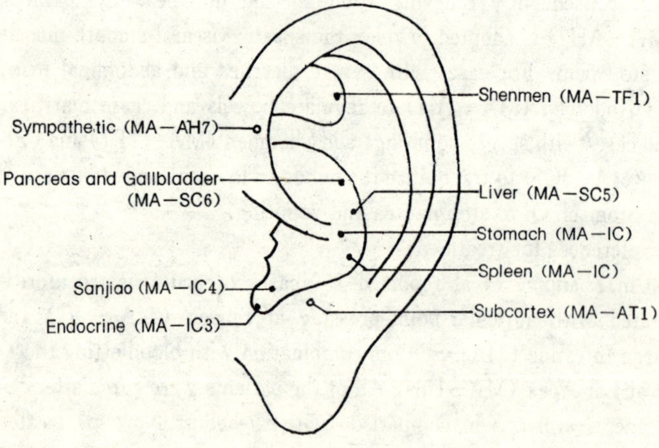

Fig. 5—9 Points for chronic gastritis

Main points: Stomach (MA—IC), Spleen (MA—IC), Shenmen

(MA－TF1), Subcortex (MA－AT1), Sympathetic (MA－AH7).

Supplementary points: Pancreas and gallbladder (MA－SC6), Endocrine (MA－IC3), Sanjiao (MA－IC4), Liver (MA－SC5).

Method: Apply auricular-point-pressing therapy with vaccaria seeds. The opposite pressing or perpendicular pressing method is recommended.

Basis for selection of point

Primary therapeutic principle should be promoting the flow of Qi to eliminate undigested food and strengthening the Spleen and Stomach. Therefore, Stomach (MA－IC) and Spleen (MA－IC) are selected to regulate gastrointestinal function. Sympathetic (MA－AH7), Shenmen (MA－TF1) and Subcortex (MA－AT1) are used to fortify the efficacy of reducing inflammation, tranquilizing the mind, relieving spasm and easing pain. For atrophic gastritis, add Pancreas and Gallbladder (MA－SC6) and Endocrine (MA－IC3). For cases with severe distension of the abdomen, add Sanjiao (MA－IC4) and Liver (MA－SC5).

References for treatment

Sun Jingsheng reported 96 cases of superficial gastritis treated mainly with auricular-point-pressing at Stomach (MA－IC), Spleen (MA－IC), Sanjiao (MA－IC4) and Liver (MA－SC5). Results: 56 cases were cured (58.3%), 28 cases were remarkably improved (29.2%), 8 cases were mildly improved (8.3%), and 4 were ineffective (4.2%). The total effective rate was 95.8%.

Wang Zhong reported 84 cases of gastritis treated mainly with auricular-point-pressing. Main points used were Stomach (MA－IC), Spleen (MA－IC) and Sympathetic (MA－AH7). Supplementary points were Pancreas and Gallbladder (MA－SC6) and Liver (MA－SC5). Results: 48 cases were cured (58.3%), 23 cases were remarkably improved (29.2%), 7 cases were mildly improved (8.3%), and 6 were ineffective (4.2%). The total effective rate was 92.8%.

10. Gastroduodenal ulcer

Gastroduodenal ulcer, also called peptic ulcer, is mostly caused by mental stress, irregular diet and dysfunction of the vegetative nervous system which lead to changes of the parietal cells in motor, secretion and nutrition. It is characterized by long-term, recurrent and episodic epigastric pain, accompanied by belching, acid regurgitation, nausea and vomiting.

In TCM, gastroduodenal ulcer belongs to the category of *Wei Wan Tong* (Epigastric Pain).

Point (Fig. 5—10) and method

Main points: Stomach (MA — IC), Duodenum (MA — SC1), Spleen (MA—IC), Sympathetic (MA—AH7), Subcortex (MA—AT1).

Supplementary points: Shenmen (MA — TF1), Liver (MA — SC5), Sanjiao (MA—IC4).

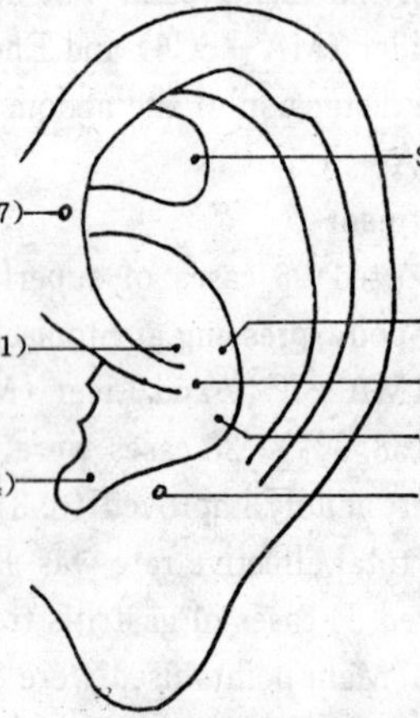

Fig. 5—10 Points for gastroduodenal ulcer

Method: Mostly apply auricular-point-pressing therapy with vaccaria seeds. The opposite pressing or perpendicular pressing method is recommended.

Basis for selection of point

Primary therapeutic principle should be promoting the flow of Qi to stop pain, easing the Stomach and strengthening the Spleen, enriching Blood and dredging Channels. Stomach (MA — IC) and

Spleen (MA—IC) are selected as the points corresponding to the diseased focus. Since the Spleen and the Stomach are exteriorly-interiorly related, Spleen (MA—IC) is used to help tonify the Spleen and the Stomach, to nourish Blood and dredge Channels to promote the healing of ulcer. Subcortex (MA—AT1) and Sympathetic (MA—AH7) are used to tranquilize the mind and relieve spasm, to promote flow of Qi and stop pain via regulating the functions of the cerebral cortex and vegetative nerve. Add Shenmen (MA—TF1) for severe pain, Liver (MA—SC5) and Sanjiao (MA—IC4) for distending pain of the epigastric region involving the hypochondrium. In case of active period with hemorrhage, deduct Sympathetic (MA—AH7) and add Ear Center (MA—H1).

References for treatment

Wang Zhong et al reported 124 cases of peptic ulcer treated with auricular puncture. Results: 32 cases were cured, 36 cases were remarkably improved, 42 cases were mildly improved, and 14 were not improved. The total effective rate was 88.6%.

Remarks

Auricular-point-pressing therapy proves quite effective for peptic ulcer and chronic gastritis, especially in alleviating symptoms and ceasing pain. However, because these diseases usually have a long duration, long-term treatment is needed to consolidate the curative effects.

11. Phrenospasm

Phrenospasm refers to the involuntary contraction of the diaphragm led by phrenic nerve being stimulated. It is mostly caused by exposure to cold or overeating, or subsequent to some digestive diseases or operation. The main manifestation is an involuntary, short, quick and frequent sound from the throat due to reversed flow of the air in the Stomach.

In TCM, phrenospasm belongs to the category of *E Ni* (Hiccup). It is considered to be caused by improper diet or emotional disturbances causing adverse rise of the Stomach Qi and further affecting the diaphragm.

Point (Fig. 5—11) and method

Points: Ear Center (MA—H1), Stomach (MA—IC), Liver (MA—SC5), Shenmen (MA—TF1), Sympathetic (MA—AH7), Subcortex (MA—AT1).

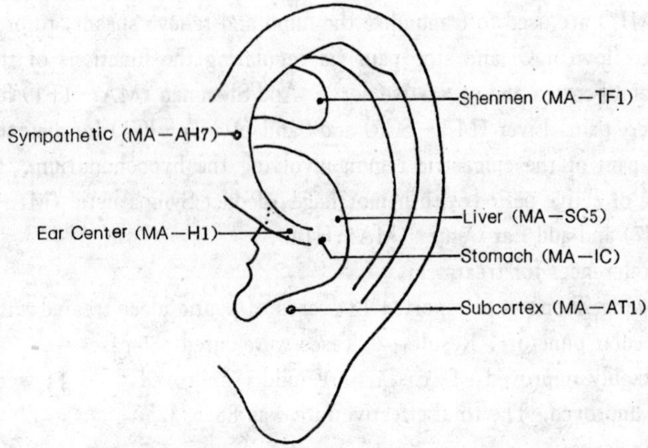

Fig. 5—11 Points for gastroptosis

Method: Mostly apply auricular-point-pressing therapy with vaccaria seeds. Strong stimulation of the opposite pressing or perpendicular pressing is recommended.

Basis for selection of point

Ear Center (MA—H1), also called Diaphragm Point, is selected to regulate Qi activities and send down the adverse rise of the Stomach Qi to stop hiccup. Stomach (MA—IC) and Liver (MA—SC5) are used in combination to regulate the Stomach, to soothe the Liver and check the adverse flow of Qi. Subcortex (MA—AT1) is used to eliminate pathological exciting focus of the cerebral cortex and regulate gastrointestinal functions, Sympathetic (MA—AH7) to alleviate spasm of the smooth muscle, Shenmen (MA—TF1) to tranquilize the mind, to relieve spasm and arrest hiccup. The joint use of the above points can regulate Qi movement and send down the adverse flow of the Stomach Qi to stop hiccup, and also reduce harmful stimulation on the cerebral cortex led by the spasm of the diaphragm, thus breaking the pathological reaction chain.

References for treatment

Liu Shulan reported 47 cases of severe hiccup treated with auricular needling. The main points used were Ear Center (MA－H1), Liver (MA－SC5), Spleen (MA－IC), Stomach (MA－IC) and Sympathetic (MA－AH7). The Supplementary points were Shenmen (MA－TF1) and Subcortex (MA－AT1). All of the patients were cured after 1－2 treatments.

12. Gastroptosis

Gastroptosis refers to the morbid condition in which the whole stomach descends to an abnormal position, namely, the lower border of the stomach reaches the pelvic cavity and the lowest point of the lesser curvature of the stomach is lower than the level of the inter-iliac-crest line. Gastroptosis is a common disease, frequently seen in those who have a thin and weak body with a long and narrow thorax, in multiparas, or in those who frequently overwork immediately after meals. The main clinical manifestations include epigastric distension, discomfort or pain with sinking sensation and belching after meals. These symptoms are aggravated by standing or fatigue while relieved by lying flat, and they are accompanied by anorexia, nausea, vomiting, palpitation, lassitude, constipation, etc. Emaciation, sallow complexion and listlessness may appear in patients with a long duration.

In TCM, gastroptosis belongs to the category of *Wei Huan* (Loosened Stomach), which is considered to be caused by deficiency of the Spleen and Stomach leading to sinking of the *Zhong Qi* (Central Qi).

Point (Fig. 5－12) and method

Main points: Spleen (MA－IC), Stomach (MA－IC), Ear Center (MA－H1), Sympathetic (MA－AH7), Subcortex (MA－AT1).

Supplementary points: Sanjiao (MA－IC4), Large Intestine (MA－SC4).

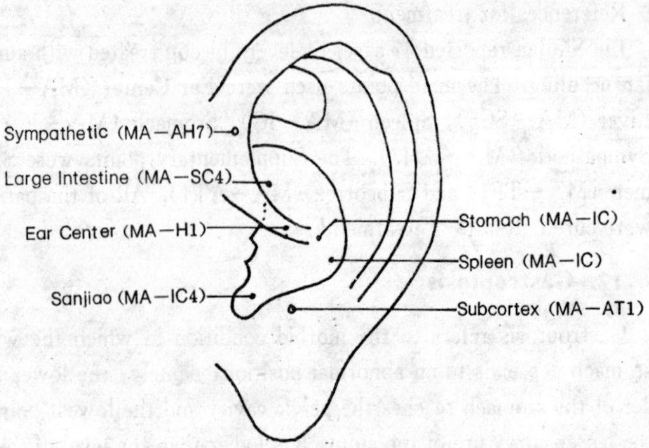

Fig. 5—12 Points for gastroptosis

Method: Apply auricular-point-pressing therapy with vaccaria seeds. The perpendicular pressing or intermittent pressing is recommended.

Basis for selection of point

Treatment should be based on tonifying the Spleen and invigorating Qi. The Spleen takes charge of transporting and transforming nutrients and controls muscles. Normally the Spleen Qi tends to ascend. Only with adequate and vigorous Qi and normal function of the Spleen can the Central Qi be forceful enough to ascend. Therefore, Spleen (MA—IC) is selected in combination with Stomach (MA—IC) to strengthen the Spleen and the Stomach and invigorate the Central Qi. Ear Center (MA—H1), Sympathetic (MA—AH7) and Subcortex (MA—AT1) are used to regulate the gastrointestinal function and strengthen the force of Qi in ascending. Add Sanjiao (MA—IC4) for anorexia and abdominal distension, and Large Intestine (MA—SC4) for constipation.

Remarks

Auricular-point-pressing therapy presents certain effectiveness in treating gastroptosis. In order to improve therapeutic effects, during the period of treatment, the patient should be instructed to perform abdominal respiration 2—3 times per day, each time lasting for 3—5 minutes. Physical exercises may be adopted in combination to help build up constitution.

13. Cholecystitis and cholelithiasis

Cholecystitis and cholelithiasis are two most common diseases in the biliary tract disorders. Cholecystitis is mostly caused by invasion of bacteria and obstruction of the biliary tract, while cholelithiasis results from infection of the biliary tract, metabolic disturbance, nervous dysfunction and cholestasis. Since cholelithiasis is frequently complicated with biliary tract infection and they are the cause and effect of each other, the two diseases are discussed together here.

Both diseases manifest themselves as pain in the right upper abdomen and right hypochondrium, which may radiate to the shoulder and back, accompanied with nausea, vomiting, aversion to greasy food, abdominal distension, constipation, bitter taste of the mouth, fever, and occasionally with jaundice. Physical examination may find positive Murphy's sign. Ultrasonic B examination can help make a definite diagnosis.

In TCM, cholecystitis and cholelithiasis belong to the category of *Xie Tong* (Hypochondriac Pain).

Point (Fig. 5—13) and method

Main points: Pancreas and Gallbladder (MA—SC6), Liver (MA—SC5), Duodenum (MA—SC1), Sympathetic (MA—AH7), Subcortex (MA—AT1), Endocrine (MA—IC3), Shenmen (MA—TF1).

Supplementary points: Sanjiao (MA—IC4), Stomach (MA—IC), Ear Apex (MA—H6), Root of Ear Vagus (MA—PS).

Method: Apply auricular-point-pressing therapy with vaccaria seeds. The opposite pressing or perpendicular pressing method is recommended. Ear Apex (MA—H1) is usually pricked to cause bleeding.

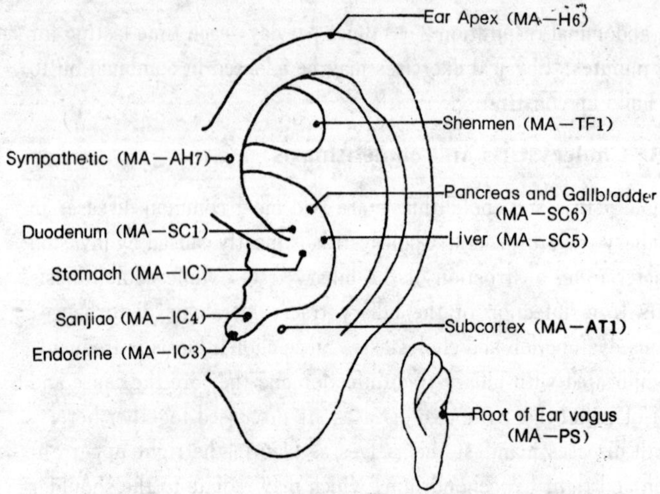

Fig. 5—13 Point for cholecystitis and cholelithiasis

Basis for selection of point

The disease should be treated with the therapeutic principle of relieving inflammation to normalize the secretion and discharge of bile and relieving spasm to stop pain. Pancreas and Gallbladder (MA—SC6), Liver (MA—SC5) and Duodenum (MA—SC1) are used to soothe the Liver and promote the function of Gallbladder, to activate the flow of Qi and alleviate mental depression, to clear away Heat and eliminate Dampness. Modern research has revealed that these three points being stimulated can promote gallbladder contraction and bile secretion. Sympathetic (MA—AH7) and Subcortex (MA—AT1) can regulate the diastolic and contractive action of the common bile duct and relieve its spasm. Endocrine (MA—IC3) and Shenmen (MA—TF1) are used to relieve inflammation and stop pain. The joint use of the above points can work in line with the therapeutic principle. For abdominal distension and constipation, Sanjiao (MA—IC4) is added to promote the flow of Qi in the Intestine and relax the bowels. For cases with nausea and vomiting, Stomach (MA—IC) is added to regulate the Stomach and send down the adverse flow of the Stomach Qi. For cases with fever, Ear Apex (MA—H6) is added to clear away Heat and remove Toxin. For cholelithiasis, Root of Ear Vagus (MA—PS) is added to help promote the function of the gallbladder in discharging calculi.

Reference for treatment

Zhao Hong reported 22 cases of cholecystitis treated with auricular- point-pressing at Pancreas and Gallbladder (MA—SC6), Liver (MA—SC5), Shenmen (MA—TF1), Spleen (MA—IC). After one course of treatment, all of the patients obtained improvement. The total effective rate was 100%.

Wang Qixiang reported 460 cases of cholecystitis and cholelithiasis treated with auricular-point-pressing therapy. The points used were: Pancreas and Gallbladder (MA—SC6), Liver (MA—SC5), Sympathetic (MA—AH7), Shenmen (MA—TF1), Subcortex (MA—AT1), Spleen (MA—IC), Sanjiao (MA—IC4) and Stomach (MA—IC). Among the cholecystitis patients (n=260) who received 10—40 treatments, 156 were cured, marked by complete disappearance of symptoms and no abnormalities found by ultrasonic B examination; 91 were improved, marked by improved symptoms and signs which were confirmed by ultrasonic B examination; and 13 were not improved. The total effective rate was 95%. Among the cholelithiasis patients (n=200) who received 1—40 treatments, 90 were cured (45%), marked by complete elimination of calculi through ultrasonic B examination and by disappearance of symptoms; 104 were improved, marked by discharge of calculi but also some others being remained in the gallbladder through ultrasonic B examination and by improvement of symptoms; and 6 were not improved.

Yang Liuchun observed the influence of auricular-point-pressing on the Gallbladder under ultrasonic B examination. Points selected were Pancreas and Gallbladder (MA—SC6), Liver (MA—SC5) and Duodenum (MA—SC1). Results showed obvious shrinkage of the gallbladder in acoustic image, especially during 5—10 minutes after treatment. There was no evident change when other irrelevant points were pressed.

Wang Xiaofu et al reported 513 cases of cholecystitis treated with combined use of three therapies including auricular-point-pressing therapy with vaccaria seeds at Pancreas and Gallbladder (MA-SC6), Shenmen (MA-TF1) and Sympathetic (MA-AH7), Pai Shi Tang (Decoction for Removing Stone) once per day, and fat meal. Results: 369 cases (71.9%) showed disappearance of symptoms and complete elimination of calculi confirmed by ultrasonic B examination or cholecystography, 134 cases (26.2%) showed improvement of symptoms and discharge of calculi but there were remained calculi found by ultrasonic B examination, and 10 cases (1.9%) showed no response. Among the 513 cases, 503 cases had discharged stones, of which 253 was bigger than 0.5 cm in diameter and the biggest was 2.5 cm.

Remarks

Auricular-point-pressing therapy proves quite effective for cholecystitis and cholelithiasis and is extensively used in clinical practice. However, attention should be paid to the following:

Symptoms of cholecystitis is often ameliorated quickly, improvement, however, displayed in ultrasonic B examination may need 1—2 months' treatment. Therefore, even though the symptoms have disappeared completely, the patient should be asked to continue the treatment for a period of time to fortify the therapeutic efficacy.

When treating cholelithiasis, to select appropriate cases is necessary. Generally, auricular-point-pressing therapy is suitable for those whose calculi are less than 10 mm in diameter and whose symptoms are obvious. If the stone is larger than 10 mm in diameter, it is difficult to be removed. This therapy is quite suitable for sand-like calculi or postoperative residual calculi.

Pay close attention to alteration of the patient's pathological condition.

If body acupuncture, herbal medicine, etc. are combined with this therapy, therapeutic effects can be improved.

Encourage the patient to have fat meal during treatment. Fat meal usually will not result in severe pain. Furthermore, it can increase appetite, ameliorate recovery of biliary function and promote bile secretion, thus facilitating discharge of calculi.

14. Chronic diarrhea

Chronic diarrhea is a common disease manifested mainly by increased frequency of stools, unformed, thin or watery feces possibly mixed with mucus, pus, blood or excessive fat. Accompanying symptoms may be abdominal pain, anorexia, sallow complexion and lassitude. The chronic diarrhea is defined as successive or recurrent diarrhea over 2 months.

Chronic diarrhea may be caused by digestive diseases, non-digestive chronic diseases or other possible reasons. The pathological changes are largely organic, but a few are functional.

In TCM, chronic diarrhea belongs to the category of *Xie Xie* (Diarrhea). It is considered to be caused mainly by improper diet and invasion of exopathogens which impair the function of the Spleen and the Stomach in transporting and transforming nutrients.

Point (Fig. 5−14) and method

Main points: Spleen (MA−IC), Stomach (MA−IC), Large Intestine (MA−SC4), Small Intestine (MA−SC2), Sympathetic (MA−AH7), Subcortex (MA−AT1).

Supplementary points: Lung (MA−IC1), Liver (MA−SC5), Kidney (MA−SC), Sanjiao (MA−IC4).

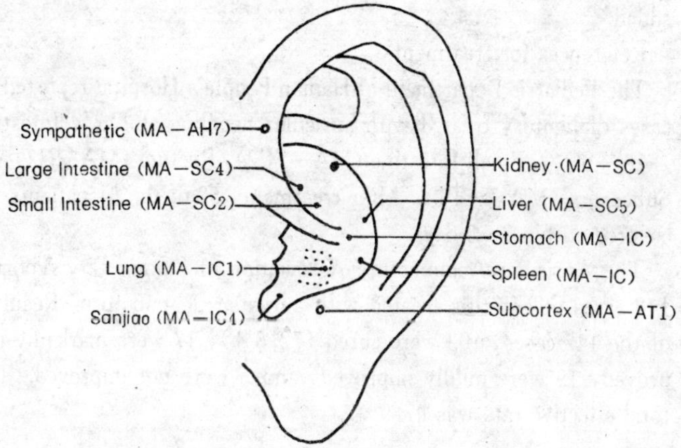

Fig. 5−14 Points for chronic diarrhea

Method: Apply auricular-point-pressing therapy with vaccaria seeds. The perpendicular pressing method is recommended. For patient with weak constitution due to long duration of diarrhea, the intermittent pressing is applied.

Basis for selection of point

The treatment is aimed at reinforcing the Spleen and the Stomach, regulating the Intestine to arrest diarrhea. Therefore, Spleen (MA—IC), Stomach (MA—IC), Large Intestine (MA—SC4) and Small Intestine (MA—SC2) are selected as the main points. Sympathetic (MA—AH7) and Subcortex (MA—AT1) are used to regulate gastrointestinal functions and relieve inflammation to arrest diarrhea. Since the Lung is interiorly-exteriorly related with the Large Intestine, Lung (MA—IC1) is supplemented to help Large Intestine (MA—SC4) increase the efficacy of regulating the Intestine to arrest diarrhea. For patients with long history of morning diarrhea accompanied with weakness of loins and legs, which is differentiated as Kidney deficiency, Kidney (MA—SC) is added. For diarrhea mixed with undigested food and much fat, which is differentiated as lientery, Sanjiao (MA—IC4) is added. For diarrhea occurring whenever the patient experiences emotional disturbances, which is differentiated as depression of the Liver Qi, Liver (MA—SC5) is added.

References for treatment

The Pediatric Department of Hainan People's Hospital reported 61 cases of lientery treated with auricular needling at Large Intestine (MA—SC4), Small Intestine (MA—SC2), Rectum (MA—H2) and Subcortex (MA—AT1). After treatment, 58 of the 61 patients recovered within 3—5 days.

The Auricular Acupuncture Association of Zigong City reported 142 cases of enteritis treated with auricular acupuncture. Results: of the 142 cases, 103 were cured (72.5%), 17 were markedly improved, 19 were mildly improved, and 3 were not improved. The total effective rate was 97.9%.

15. Constipation

Constipation, a common clinical symptom, refers to a morbid condition in which bowels is decreased in frequency, discharged with difficulty, and changed in form. For healthy people, the frequency of bowels may be quite different because of different life style and dietary habit. However, most adults evacuate bowels once every day or every other day. If a person has not evacuated bowels over 48 hours, accompanied with discomfort feeling, this condition can be considered as constipation.

Constipation manifests itself mainly by dry and hard stools and being difficult to discharge, accompanied by abdominal pain or distension, possible headache, dizziness, anorexia, nausea, vomiting, palpitation and fatigue.

In *Shang Han Za Bin Lun* (Treatise on Febrile Diseases), constipation is termed as *Yang Jie* (Yang Constipation), *Yin Jie* (Yin Constipation), *Pi Jie* (Spleen Constipation), etc. As a collective term in modern TCM, constipation is divided into two types: ① The deficiency type, which is frequently encountered in postpartum, elderly and weak people because of deficiency of Qi and Blood and consumption of the Kidney Essence; and ② The excess type, which is mostly caused by improper diet, over intake of pungent food, or febrile diseases leading to exhaustion of Body Fluid.

Point (Fig. 5−15) and method

Main points: Rectum (MA−H2), Large Intestine (MA−SC4), Constipation Point (MA), Sanjiao (MA−IC4), Lung (MA−IC1).

Supplementary points: Spleen (MA − IC), Endocrine (MA − IC3), Ear Apex (MA−H6), Stomach (MA−IC).

Method: Apply auricular-point-pressing therapy with vaccaria seeds or magnetic beads. The perpendicular pressing is suitable for the excessive type, and the intermittent pressing is suitable for the deficiency type.

Basis for selection of points

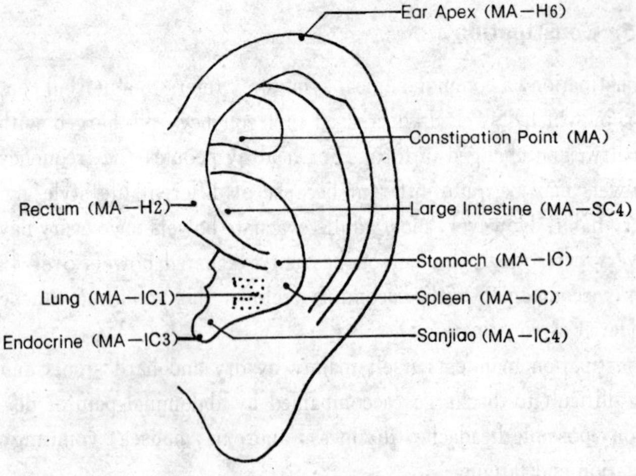

Fig. 5-15 Points for constipation

The treatment is aimed at regulating the Intestine. Rectum (MA-H2) and Large Intestine (MA-SC4) can promote the intestinal peristalsis, and send down the Qi of the Fu organs to release the bowels. Constipation Point (MA), an empirical point, has the function of moistening the Intestine and relaxing the bowels. Sanjiao (MA-IC4) being stimulated can transform Qi and transport Essence to facilitate defecation. The Lung and the Large Intestine are interiorly-exteriorly related, Lung (MA-IC1) is therefore selected to help Large Intestine (MA-SC4) with its efficacy of activating the flow of Qi to remove the feces. For the deficiency type, Spleen (MA-IC) and Endocrine (MA-IC3) are added to invigorate Qi by reinforcing the Spleen, and moisten dryness by enriching Blood. For the excess type, Ear Apex (MA-H6) and Stomach (MA-IC) are added to clear away Heat from the Yangming Channel to relax stools.

References for treatment

Song Junhui et al reported 53 cases of constipation treated with auricular-point-pressing with vaccaria seeds. Among the patients, the longest duration was 10 years while the shortest 2 weeks. Main points used were: Large Intestine (MA-SC4), Rectum (MA-

H2), Abdomen (MA－AH), Center of Superior concha (MA－SC). Supplementary points were: Spleen (MA－IC) and Stomach (MA－IC) for the deficiency type, and Sanjiao (MA－IC4) and Lung (MA－IC1) for the excess type. Results: after 5 treatments 12 cases were cured, marked by normal defecation which was maintained for at least two months after the treatment was discontinued; 24 cases were remarkably improved, marked by normal defecation; however, the patient suffered from relapse within two months after the treatment was discontinued; and 12 cases were mildly improved, marked by normal defecation, however, the patient suffered from relapse three days later after treatment was discontinued. The total effective rate was 90.5%.

Pan Jihua reported 134 cases of constipation treated with auricular-point-pressing with vaccaria seeds, of which the longest history was 16 years while the shortest 7 days. Main points selected were: Large Intestine (MA－SC4), Rectum (MA－H2), Constipation Point (MA). Supplementary points were: Ear Apex (MA－H6) and Adrenal Gland (MA－T) for the Heat type; Spleen (MA－IC) and Kidney (MA－SC) for the deficiency type. Treatment was carried out once every other day with alternate use of the two ears. One therapeutic course consists of seven sessions. Of the 134 cases, 93 cases were cured, marked by normal defecation (once daily) and disappearance of accompanying symptoms which did not recur for half a year; 29 cases were remarkably improved, marked by normal defecation, disappearance and no recurrence of most accompanying symptoms for half a year; 7 were mildly improved, marked by nearly normal defecation (once every other day) and partial improvement of accompanying symptoms; and 5 were not improved. The total effective rate was 96.3% and cure rate was 69%. The treatments ranged from 2－16 times, mean 7.

Remarks

Auricular points present significant effects for constipation. For those sensitive to this therapy, pressing the points concerned with fingers can relieve constipation. For those suffering from habitual constipation, although remarkable effects or temporary recovery are achieved, persistent treatment with finger pressing or massage at auricular points 1—2 times daily is recommended to consolidate the effects or prevent recurrence.

16. Diabetes mellitus

Diabetes mellitus is a chronic metabolic disease determined by hereditary genes. Its main pathological change is disturbance of carbohydrate, fat and protein due to relative or absolute insufficiency of insulin. The major characteristics are hyperglycemia and glycuresis. In early stage, symptoms may not present. However, polyuria, polyphagia, polydipsia, emaciation and fatigue will emerge with the development of disease. In severe cases, ketoacidosis may occur.

In TCM, diabetes mellitus belongs to the categories of *Xiao Ke* (Serious Thirst, or Diabetes). According to different characteristics of clinical symptoms, it is classified into three types: ① *Shang Xiao* (Upper Diabetes), which is basically associated with the Lung and manifested by hot sensation in the throat, unbearable thirst and polydipsia; ② *Zhong Xiao* (Middle Diabetes), which is basically associated with the Stomach and manifested by pholyphagia, insatiable hunger, spontaneous perspiration, emaciation and dry stools; and ③ *Xia Xiao* (Lower Diabetes), which is basically associated with the Kidney and manifested by frequent, excessive and turbid urination with sweet smell. These three types or two of them may develop simultaneously. Seldom does the upper diabetes exists alone.

Point (Fig. 5—16) and method

Main points: Pancreas and Gallbladder (MA—SC6), Pancreasitis Point (MA), Sanjiao (MA—IC4), Endocrine (MA—IC3), Central Rim (MA—AT).

Supplementary points: Lung (MA—IC1), Thirst Point (MA), Spleen (MA—IC), Stomach (MA—IC), Hunger Point (MA), Kidney (MA—SC).

Method: Apply auricular-point-pressing therapy with vaccaria seeds or magnetic beads. The perpendicular pressing or the intermittent pressing or recommended.

Basis for selection of points

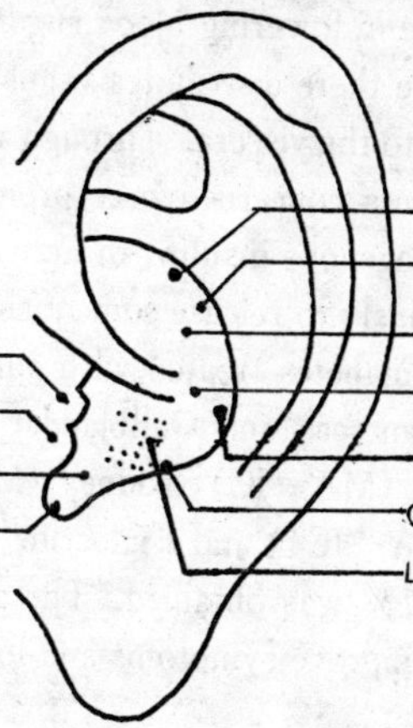

Fig. 5—16 Points for diabetes mellitus

As the corresponding point to the diseased area, Pancreas and Gallbladder (MA—SC6) is selected. Pancreasitis Point (MA) is an empirical point for diabetes. Both points have the function of regulating the pancreas. Sanjiao (MA — IC4) is used to regulate Qi movement, smooth the Sanjiao and clear away stagnated Heat there. Endocrine (MA—IC3) and Central Rim (MA—AT) are selected to promote secretion of insulin by regulating visceral and endocrine function, thus reducing blood sugar.

For polydipsia, add Lung (MA—IC1) and Thirst Point (MA) to clear away Heat from the Lung and nourish Yin to relieve thirst. For polyphagia, add Spleen (MA—IC) and Hunger Point (MA) to clear away Stomach Heat and invigorate the Spleen to distribute Body Fluid. For polyuria, add Kidney (MA—SC) to nourish Yin, to tonify the Kidney and conserve Essence.

References for treatment

Long Wenjun reported 25 cases of diabetes treated with auricular needling mainly at Pancreas and Gallbladder (MA—SC6), Central Rim (MA—AT), Endocrine (MA—IC3), Kidney (MA—SC) and Sanjiao (MA — IC4). Results revealed a significant change of the blood sugar after treatment ($P<0.001$). This indicated that auricular points are effective in lowering blood sugar. The author pointed out that on the auricle there distributes vagus nerve on most of the points corresponding to the viscera. Through vagus nerve, stimulating the auricular points concerned may promote pancreatic island cells B to secrete endogenous insulin, or activate those without secretary function previously to release some insulin. Yang Lanxu et al reported 60 cases of diabetes treated with auricular- point-pressing therapy mainly at Pancreas and Gallbladder (MA — SC6), Liver (MA—SC5), Spleen (MA—IC), Kidney (MA—SC), Lung (MA — IC1), Sanjiao (MA—IC4) and Endocrine (MA—IC3). A total effective rate of 86.7% was obtained. The author considered that auricular points can improve symptoms and lower blood sugar.

Remarks

Auricular points prove effective for diabetes in improving subjective symptoms and reducing glucose in blood and urine. For IDDM patients, only when subjective symptoms have improved and blood sugar has reduced or approximated to normal can the dosage of insulin be decreased.

Patients should be asked to adjust diet and do appropriate physical exercises while receiving auricular pressing treatment.

Since patients with diabetes are susceptible to infection, it is asked to sterilize carefully, to press gently, and to retain the seeds not too long (2—3 days is proper).

17. Obesity

Obesity refers to excessive fat of the body. It can be classified as simple and secondary types. Generally obesity denotes the simple type, which is defined as 20% over the standard weight, excluding those due to water-sodium retention and excessive muscles.

Simple obesity can be caused by harmful dietary habit or life style, lack of activity during recuperation after illness, genetic, neuropsychological or endocrine factors. It may develop at any age but more common in middle-aged females. Simple obesity is usually asymptomatic; in severe cases, however, it may present dizziness, headache, fatigue, depression and hypogonadism.

1) Formula for calculating standard weight (Broca's)

For those taller than 150 cm

Standard weight (kg) =[height(cm)−100]×0.9

For those shorter than 150 cm

Standard weight (kg) = height(cm)−100

2) Evaluation of overweight

Obesity scale = (actual weight − standard weight)÷ standard weight×100%

The actual weight that surpasses the standard weight by 10%-19% is defined as overweight; by 20% above, obesity; by 20%-30%, mild obesity, by 30%-50%, moderate obesity; and by 50% above, severe obesity.

In TCM, obesity is mainly discussed in *Qi Xu* (Qi Deficiency) and *Tan Yin* (Stagnation of Phlegm and Dampness).

Point (Fig. 5−17) and method

Main points: Spleen (MA−IC), Stomach (MA−IC), Sanjiao (MA−IC4), Endocrine (MA−IC3), Subcortex (MA−AT1), Sympathetic (MA−AT7), Hunger Point (MA).

Supplementary points: Points corresponding to the fat-stagnated areas, Kidney (MA−SC).

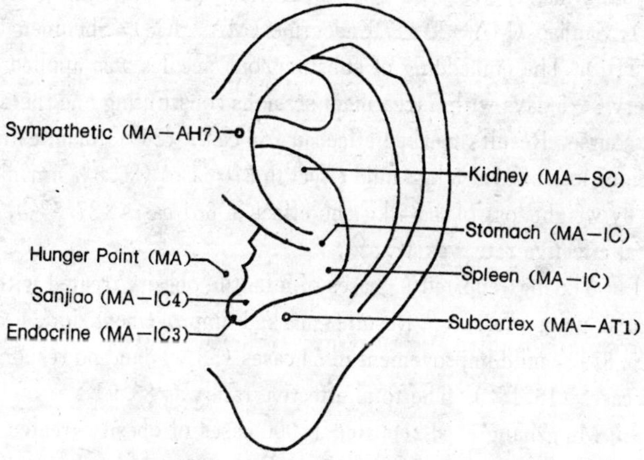

Fig. 5−17 Points for obesity

Method: Apply auricular-point-pressing therapy with vaccaria seeds. The opposite pressing or perpendicular pressing is recommended.

Basis for selection of point

TCM holds that fat people have excessive Phlegm and Dampness. Therefore, the treatment is aimed to strengthen the Spleen, to invigorate Qi, to dispel Phlegm and resolve Dampness, and for these purposes Spleen (MA—IC), Stomach (MA—IC) and Sanjiao (MA—IC4) are selected. Based on Western medicine, Endocrine (MA—IC3), Subcortex (MA—AT1), Sympathetic (MA—AT7) and Hunger Point (MA) are selected to regulate the action of the viscera and endocrine system, to exeite the appetite regulatory center, and to enhance sympathetic excitability, thus promoting the decomposition of fat to reduce its accumulation and inducing a sensation of fullness to decrease intake of food. Fat is reduced as a result.

According to different area where fat is accumulated, Neck (MA—AH7) and/or Abdomen (MA—AH) can be treated at. If the patient has edema, Kidney (MA—SC) is added to promote urination.

References for treatment

Cui Shugui reported 1015 cases of obesity treated with auricular needling mainly at Large Intestine (MA—SC4), Stomach (MA—IC), Sanjiao (MA—IC4), Endocrine (MA—IC3), Shenmen (MA—TF1). The embedding of subcutaneous needles was applied once every 3—5 days with 5 treatment sessions constituting one therapeutic course. Result: marked effect in 264 cases (26%) manifested by weight loss of over 5 kg; mild effect in 370 cases (36.5%) manifested by weight loss of 3—5 kg; no effect in 381 cases (37.5%). The total effective rate was 62.5%.

Liu Yixiang reported 93 cases of infantile obesity treated with auricular-point-pressing. Result: marked improvement in 24 cases (25.8%), mild improvement in 54 cases (58%), and no response in 15 cases (16.1%). The total effective rate was 83.9%.

Lu Mingzhang et al reported 1,000 cases of obesity treated with pressing of vaccaria seeds mainly at Endocrine (MA—IC3), Stomach (MA—IC), Mouth (MA—IC5) and Hunger Point (MA). The seeds were changed every 2—3 days with 10 treatment constituting one course. After one treatment course, 448 cases obtained 2.5 kg of weight loss, 353 cases obtained 1.4—2.4 kg of weight loss, and 199 cases had no response. The total effective rate was 80.1%.

Remarks

Auricular points prove quite effective for simple obesity. However, a rather long period of treatment, generally 1—2 months, is required. Clinical observation shows that most patients obtain 1—3 kg of weight loss after 1—2 treatment courses. The weight may not reduce or even increase during a period of successive treatments. However, if the treatment is continued, the weight may reduce gradually again. Therefore, persistent treatment is important for reducing weight.

The treatment is suitable for the simple obesity patient with the weight surpassing the standard by 20% above. It is not suitable for those with substandard weight, for anorexia nervosa may be induced.

Discontinue the treatment after the weight has reduced to a certain level. The patient can perform massage or finger-pressing on relevant auricular points to stabilize the curative effects.

18. Hyperlipemia

Hyperlipemia refers that the plasma lipid concentration surpasses the higher limit of normal value. Blood lipid is a collective term for various plasma or serum lipids, including many fat-soluble substances. Its main components are cholesterol (CH), triglyceride (TG), phospholipid (PL) and free fatty-acid (FA). Since plasma lipid is fat-soluble and it must combine with protein to form a water-soluble compound and then can be transported to the whole body, hyperlipemia is also called hyperlipoproteinemia. Hyperlipemia is closely related with arterial athrosclerosis, diabetes, fatty liver and kidney disorders, especially cerebrovascular and cardiovascular diseases. Therefore, overcoming hyperlipemia is of great significance for people's health.

In TCM, hypelipemia belongs to the categories of *Tan Shi*

(Phlegm- Dampness) and *Fei Pang* (Obesity) and *Shi Re* (Dampness-Heat).

Point (Fig. 5—18) and method

Main points: Pancreas and Gallbladder (MA—SC6), Small Intestine (MA—IC2), Sanjiao (MA—IC4), Liver (MA—SC5), Angle of Superior Concha (MA—SC), Endocrine (MA—IC3), Spleen (MA—IC).

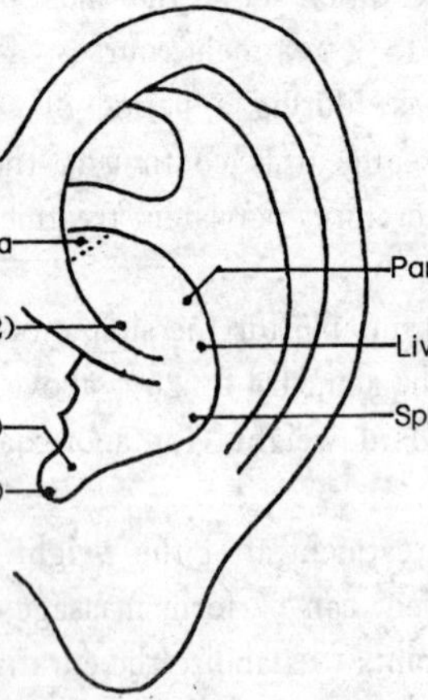

Fig. 5—18 Points for hyperlipemin

Method: Apply auricular-point-pressing with vaccaria seeds or magnetic beads. Plaster-sticking with *Xian Gui Hou Xu Gao* (Plaster for Promoting Blood Circulation with Moschus and Cortex Cinnamomi) can also be used. Opposite or perpendicular pressing with strong force is recommended for stimulating the points.

Basis for selection of point

Pancreas and Gallbladder (MA—SC6), Small Intestine (MA—IC2), Sanjiao (MA—IC4), Liver (MA—SC5) and Prostate (MA) are used to clear away Heat and Dampness, to reinforce the Middle Jiao to benefit digestion, and to promote flow of Qi to remove Blood stasis. Clinical study has revealed that Pancreas and Gallbladder (MA—SC6) has the efficacy of antilipodieresis function, marked by increasing cell's intake of fatty-acid, inhibiting lipodieresis and lowering the function of free fatty-acid in blood. Angle of Superior Concha (MA-SC) can also inhibit lipodieresis and reduce blood-lipid. Endocrine (MA-IC3) and Spleen (MA-IC) are combined with the above points to strengthen the function of eliminating Phlegm and Dampness and removing Blood stasis.

References for treatment

Yu Peng reported 523 cases of hyperlipemia treated with auricular-point-pressing. The plaster of *She Xiang Zhuang Gu Gao* (Plaster for Strengthening Bone Mainly with Moschus) and vaccaria seeds were used for pressing. The seeds were changed every 2-3 days with one therapeutic course lasting for 1 month. After treatment, cholesterol and triglyceride decreased obviously. Statistical analysis showed a significant decrease of blood-lipid after treatment ($P<0.01$).

19. Hyperthyroidism

Hyperthyroidism, one of the common diseases in endocrine system, results from excessive secretion of thyroid hormones due to various reasons. Mental stimulation and acute infection may cause dysfunction of the central nervous system leading to hypersecretion of thyroid glands via hypothalamus or pituitary. It manifests itself mainly by high metabolic symptoms, nervous hyperexcitation, general swelling of the thyroid gland and exophthalmos. The main symptoms are irritability, hyperorexia, emaciation, aversion to Heat, profuse perspiration, palpitation and exophythalmos. Basal metabolic rate rises in most cases, with the exception of a few patients.

In TCM, hyperthyroidism belongs to the category of *Ying Liu* (Goiter).

Point (Fig. 5-19) and method

Main points: Cervical Vertebrae (MA-AH8), Endocrine (MA-IC3), Central Rim (MA-AT), Subcortex (MA-AT1).

Supplementary points: Heart (MA-IC), Shenmen (MA-TF1), Hunger Point (MA), Liver (MA-SC5), Kidney (MA-SC), Sympathetic (MA-AH7).

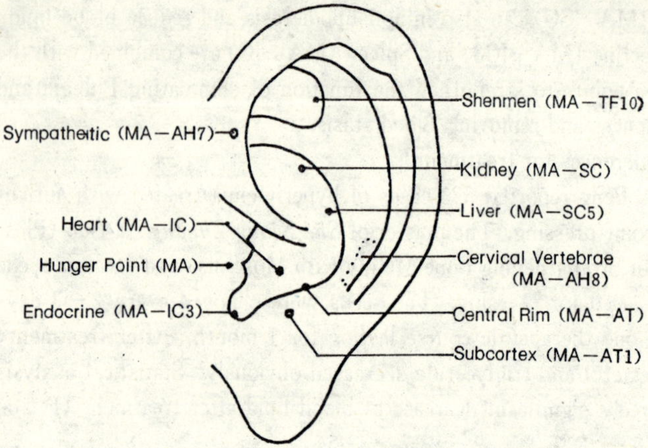

Fig. 5—19 Points for hyperthyroidism

Method: Apply auricular-point-pressing with vaccaria seeds or magnetic beads. The perpendicular pressing is recommended.

Basis for selection of point

As a point corresponding to the diseased area, Cervical Vertebrae (MA — AH8) is selected to relieve the depressed Liver, to clear away Phlegm and regulate the function of the thyroid gland. Endocrine (MA—IC3), Central Rim (MA—AT) and Subcortex (MA — AT1) are used to regulate the cerebral cortex and the pituitary gland to inhibit the secretion of thyroid hormones. Add Heart (MA —IC), Shenmen (MA—TF1) and Liver (MA—SC5) for irritability, Hunger Point (MA) for hyperorexia, and Kidney (MA—SC) and Sympathetic (MA—AH7) for aversion to heat and profuse perspiration.

Remarks

Auricular-point-pressing therapy is effective for hyperthyroidism. It can improve clinical symptoms and long-term treatment can lower basal metabolic rate.

Ask the patient to avoid emotional irritation and pay attention to diet.

20. Impotence

Impotence is an abnormal manifestation of sexual function in prematurely senile males, marked by inability to erect the penis or the hardiness of the penis being not enough to complete sexual activities when the patient is sexually stimulated or has desire for sexual life.

In addition to organic pathological change of the genitals, genital deformation, nervous injury and damage of penile cavernous muscle, impotence is mostly caused by increased inhibition of the cortex on the penis erecting or dysfunction of the spinal cord.

In TCM, this disorder is also called *Yang Wei* or *Yin Wei* (Impotence). The causes are believed to be early marriage, intemperance of sexual life, or juvenile masturbation which leads to decline of the *Ming Huo* (Vital Gate-Fire) and deficiency of the Kidney Qi, anxiety or depression which impairs the Heart and Spleen, and downward flow of Dampness-Heat which causes looseness of the penis.

Point (Fig. 5—20) and method

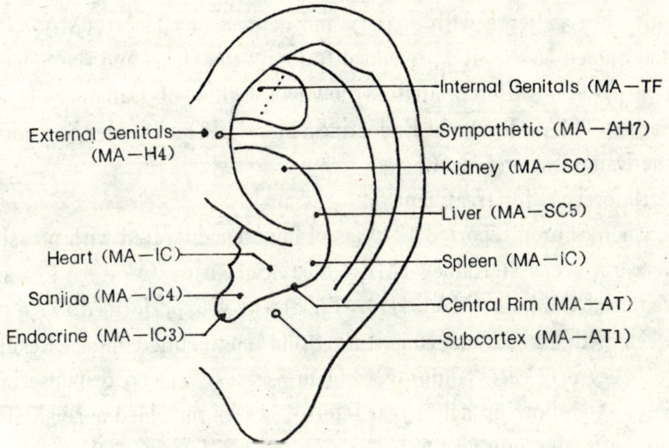

Fig. 5—20 Points for impotence

Main points: Internal Genitals (MA—TF), External Genitals (MA—H4), Kidney (MA—SC); Liver (MA—SC5), Sympathetic (MA—AH7), Subcortex (MA—AT1), Central Rim (MA—AT).

Supplementary points: Heart (MA－IC), Spleen (MA－IC), Sanjiao (MA－IC4), Endocrine (MA－IC3).

Method: Apply auricular-point-pressing with vaccaria seeds. Perpendicular or opposite pressing is recommended.

Basis for selection of point

The treatment should be aimed at tonifying the Kidney and replenishing the vital Essence to strengthen the penis. Internal Genitals (MA－TF) and External Genitals (MA－H4) are selected as the corresponding points to the focus. Since the Kidney stores the vital Essence and controls reproduction and the Liver stores Blood and controls the penis, Kidney (MA－SC) and Liver (MA－SC5) are employed to reinforce the Kidney and nourish the penis. According to modern medicine, Sympathetic (MA－AH7), Subcortex (MA－AT1) and Central Rim (MA－AT) can regulate the vegetative nervous function and relieve cortical inhibition to induce erection of the penis. The joint use of the above points can reach the purpose of tonifying the Kidney and replenishing the vital Essence to strengthen the penis. The ability of erection can be restored as a result. For patients with anxiety and depression, Heart (MA－IC) and Spleen (MA－IC) are added to tonify the Heart and the Spleen. For patients differentiated as downward flow of Dampness-Heat, Sanjiao (MA－IC4) and Endocrine (MA－IC3) are added to remove the Dampness and Heat.

References for treatment

Chen Shuren reported 13 cases of impotence treated with pressing vaccaria seeds at Kidney (MA－SC), Subcortex (MA－AT1) and External Genitals (MA－H4). Treatment was performed twice per week with 10 sessions constituting one therapeutic course. Result: recovery in 7 cases, improvement in 5 cases, and no response in 1 case. At follow-up half a year later, 10 cases remained normal. The total effective rate was 92%.

Remarks

Auricular points prove quite effective for impotence. For those sensitive to this therapy, the ability of penis erection may be restored after only one treatment.

Because impotence is mostly caused by increased inhibition of the cerebral cortex or dysfunction of the spinal center due to mental stress, anxiety and fear, removing the patient's worries and helping establish the patient's confidence is improvement to successful treatment.

21. Seminal emission

Seminal emission refers to the involuntary seminal discharge in adult males. Specifically, nocturnal emission occurs during dream more than twice per weak, while spermatorrhea happens on just a slight sexual touch and without dream at any time during day and night. However, occasional emission in young adults without any other symptoms is not considered as an abnormal condition but as the spontaneous overflow of profuse seminal fluid.

In Western medicine, spermatorrhea is considered to be caused mostly by fullness of the urinary bladder and rectum, oppression on the lower abdomen during sleep and mental stimulation. Therefore, it is believed as a functional disorder.

In TCM, nocturnal emission results from over consumption of the Kidney Yin with excess of the Heart Fire and downward flow of Dampness- Heat leading to disturbance of the sperm house, while spermatorrhea results from failure of the Kidney in controlling sperms as a result of lingering diseases. The former is an excess syndrome in most cases while the latter a deficiency syndrome.

Point (Fig. 5—21) and method

Main points: Kidney (MA—SC), Heart (MA—IC), Internal Genitals (MA), Subcortex (MA—AT1).

Supplementary points: Anterior Ear lobe (MA—L), Spleen (MA—IC), Sanjiao (MA—IC4), Central Rim (MA—AT), Endocrine (MA—IC3).

Method: Apply auricular-point-pressing therapy with vaccaria seeds. The perpendicular pressing is recommended. For deficiency syndrome, the intermittent pressing is suitable.

Basis for selection of point

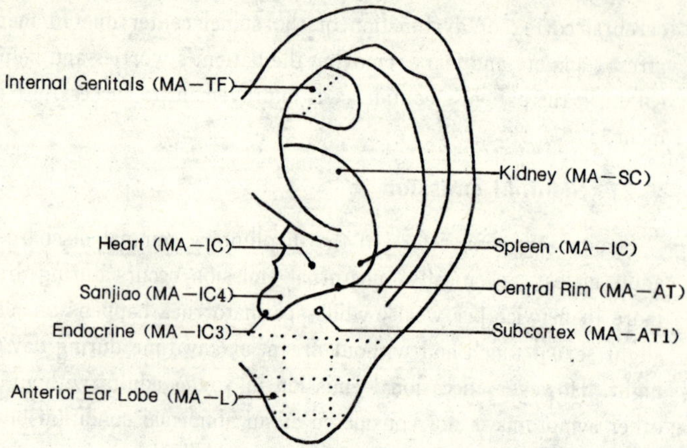

Fig. 5－21 Points for sominal emission

This disease should be treated mainly by regulating the function of the Zang-Fu organs, and astringing sperms to stop emission. According to the *Zang Xiang Xue Shuo* (Viscera-State Doctrine), the Kidney, as the foundation of native construction and the origin of the primary Yin and Yang, stores the vital Essence and generates Marrow. Therefore, Kidney (MA－SC) is selected to invigorate the Kidney Qi and nourish Yin to consolidate sperms. Heart (MA－IC) is used to send down the flared Heart Fire and calm the mind. Combined use of these two points can restore the harmony between the Heart and the Kidney by nourishing Yin and reducing Fire. Subcortex (MA－AT1) can regulate the excito-inhibitory action of the cerebral cortex. Internal Genitals (MA) is used to replenish Yang and Essence and regulate Blood. The joint use of the above points can reach the purpose of regulating the Kidney and calming the Heart, astringing sperms and stopping emission. For nocturnal emission, Shenmen (MA－TF1) and Anterior Ear Lobe (MA－L) are added to tranquilize the mind. For syndrome due to Dampness-Heat in the Lower Jiao, Liver (MA－SC5), Sanjiao (MA－IC4) and Spleen (MA－IC) are added to clear it away. For spermatorrhea, Central Rim (MA－AT) and Endocrine (MA－AH7) are added to tonify the Kidney and consolidate sperms.

Remarks

Auricular-point-pressing therapy is effective for seminal emission, especially for nocturnal emission.

Since the disease is mostly functional, it is necessary to help the patient harmonize emotions and dispel misgivings during treatment.

Ask the patient to cultivate good habits in daily life and avoid intemperance of sexual life so as to decrease the cortical excitation. Tight underclothes are inappropriate, for they can abrade the pudendum, leading to congestion of the penis and inducing spermatorrhea.

22. Enuresis

Enuresis refers to the involuntary discharge of urine though the function of urination is normal. Enuresis is characterized by micturition once or several times per night during sleep without awareness of the patient until he wakes up. Prolonged illness may bring about listlessness, poor appetite, sallow complexion and emaciation. Enuresis mostly occurs in children, occasionally in adults with intermittent sleep at night.

Enuresis results mainly from incomplete development of the higher central nervous system in controlling urination, or failure of the cerebral cortex in inhibiting the reflex contraction of the Bladder.

In TCM, the same term is used. It is considered to be caused by deficiency of the Kidney Qi failing to consolidate the Lower Jiao or by flaming up of the Fire in the Liver and Gallbladder.

Point (Fig. 5—22) and method

Main points: Kidney (MA—SC), Bladder (MA—SC8), Subcortex MA—AT1), Urethra (MA—H3).

Supplementary points: Excitation Point (MA), Liver (MA—SC5).

Method: Apply auricular-point-pressing therapy with vaccaria seeds. Finger-pressing may be used for children. The perpendicular or intermittent pressing approach is frequently adopted.

Basis for selection of point

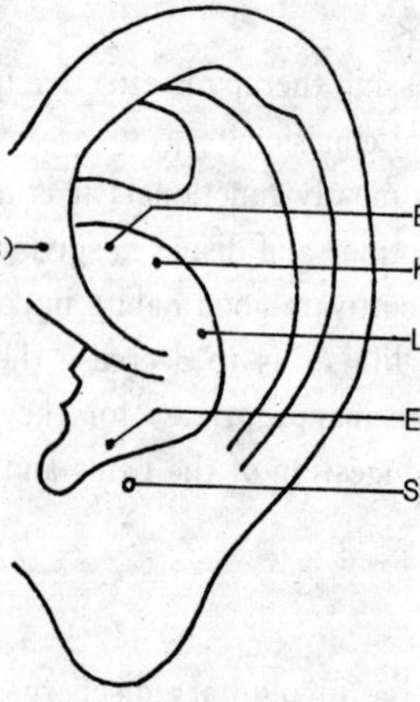

Fig. 5—22 Points for enuresis

This disease should be treated mainly with the therapeutic principle of tonifying the Kidney Qi. Kidney (MA — SC) and Bladder (MA—SC8) are used to replenish the Kidney Qi and control urination. Modern research has revealed that stimulating the above two points can regulate the function of the kidney and urinary bladder. Subcortex (MA—AT1) can strengthen the inhibitory action of the cerebral cortex on the micturition reflex. By promoting Blood circulation and dredging Channels, Urethra (MA—H3) is used to enhance the self-restraint of the urethra. The joint use of the above points can reach the aim of reinforcing the Kidney and ceasing enuresis. For children patients who cannot be easily woken up from a profound sleep, Excitation Point (MA) is added to increase the excitability of the cortical waking center. For patients differentiated symptomatically as the flaring up of the Fire in the Liver and Gallbladder, Liver (MA—SC5) is added to clear away the Fire and reinforce the Kidney Qi.

References for treatment

Wang Qijun et al reported 103 cases of enuresis treated with auricular- point-pressing therapy. Among the patients, the eldest was 17 years and the youngest 4 years. Main points used were: Kidney

(MA−SC), Bladder (MA−SC8), Urethra (MA−H3), Excitation Point (MA), Endocrine (MA−IC3). Vaccaria seeds were used to press the points and seeds were changed once every 3 days. Result: cured in 16 cases, marked by normal urination without recurrence during half a year follow-up; remarkably improved in 54 cases, marked by no enuresis after 5 treatments, however, there were occasional recurrence during half a year follow-up; mildly effective in 29 cases, marked by reduced frequency of enuresis, and ineffective in 4 cases. The total effective rate was 96.1%.

Yuan Shiyu et al reported 940 cases of enuresis treated with auricular therapy. The patients were treated with auricular-point-pressing therapy at the points selected on the basis of syndrome identification or the points selected on the basis of detection, or treated with needle-embedding therapy at the points selected on the basis of syndrome identification. Result: cured in 158 cases, remarkably improved in 229 cases, mildly effective in 480 cases, and ineffective in 73 cases. The total effective rate was 92.2%. Analysis of the results showed that all the methods used were quite effective and there were no significant difference between them ($P>0.05$).

Remarks

Auricular-point-pressing therapy proves quite effective for enuresis, especially for that in children. In the beginning of treatment, the patients are asked to wake up the affected child at certain time to urinate once or twice every night so that the child can develop a conditional reflex, which is helpful in improving therapeutic efficacy.

With auricular therapy, enuresis can be cured or remarkably improved within one treatment course generally. However, one more course of treatment is necessary to consolidate the result.

23. Frequent micturition

Frequent micturition is a common symptom in the urinary disease, defined as obvious increase of urination frequency, usually more than 3 times at night and over 5 times during the day. Too frequent urination will disturb the sleep.

In TCM, this disease is considered to be caused mostly by deficiency of the Kidney or downward flow of Dampness-Heat.

Point (Fig. 5—23) and method

Main points: Urethra (MA—H3), Kidney (MA—SC), Bladder (MA—SC8), Central Rim (MA—AT), Subcortex (MA—AT1).

Supplementary points: Occiput (MA—AT), Endocrine (MA—IC3), Liver (MA—SC5), Sanjiao (MA—IC4).

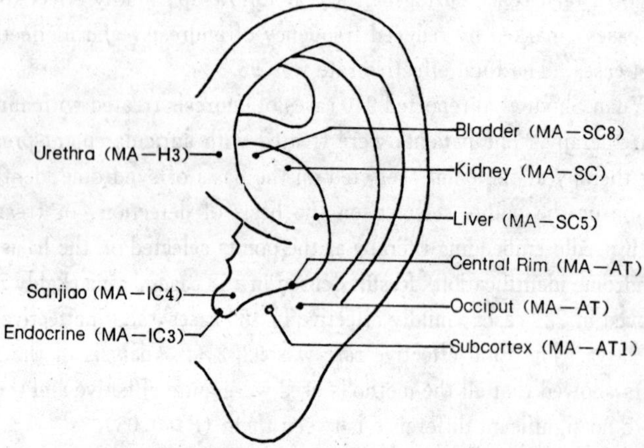

Fig. 5—23 Points for frequent micturition

Method: Apply auricular-point-pressing therapy with vaccaria seeds or magnetic beads. The perpendicular pressing or intermittent pressing approach is recommended.

Basis for selection of point

As the corresponding points to the diseased part, Urethra (MA—H3) and Bladder (MA—SC8) are selected to regulate the urinary bladder and strengthen its self-restraint action. Kidney (MA—IC) is used to reinforce the Kidney Qi and increase its protective action on the primary Qi in the Lower Jiao. Central Rim (MA—AT) and Subcortex (MA—AT1) are employed to regulate the function of the cerebral cortex and enhance its action of antidiuresis. For severe cases suffering from nocturnal frequent micturition, Occiput (MA—AT) and Endocrine (MA—IC3) are added. For those having Dampness-Heat syndrome, Liver (MA—SC5) and Sanjiao (MA—IC4) are added.

Reference for treatment

Xu Ruizheng et al reported 15 cases of frequent micturition treated with auricular-point-pressing therapy. Result: cured in 5 cases, improved in 5 cases, and ineffective in 2 cases.

Remarks

Auricular-point-pressing therapy proves quite effective for various frequent micturition. During the treatment, the patient should be asked to distract his attention from urination as far as possible.

24. Headache

Headache results from stimulation on the intracranial or extracranial pain-sensitive tissues. It is a common clinical symptom frequently seen in a variety of acute or chronic diseases. Basically, it is classified into two categories: organic and functional. To avoid misdiagnosis, attention should be paid to case history and examination.

Headache discussed here refers to those developing as a principal symptom in the internal diseases. It does not include those resulting from acute infection, diseases of the eye, ear, nose and throat, and intracranial space-occupying lesion, for which the primary disorder should be treated.

In TCM, it is in the category of *Tou Tong* (Headache). TCM holds that the head is the confluence of all the Yang Channels. According to the Channel Identification, different parts of the headache is termed after the corresponding Channels, namely, the frontal headache, temporal headache, occipital headache and parietal headache are termed respectively as the Yangming headache, Shaoyang headache, Taiyang headache and Jueyin headache. Most headaches belong to the excess syndrome, manifested by severe pain which may be a distending pain, jumping pain, or stabbing pain. Some other headaches belong to the deficiency syndrome, manifested by mild and lingering pain accompanied with dizziness, pallor complexion and listlessness.

Point (Fig. 5—24) and method

Main points: Points corresponding to the diseased part such as Forehead (MA－AT), Occiput (MA－AT) and Temple (MA－

AT), Subcortex (Ma—AT1), Sympathetic (MA—AH7), Shenmen (MA—TF1).

Supplementary points: Stomach (MA—IC), Gallbladder (MA—SC6), Bladder (MA—SC8), Liver (MA—SC5), Spleen (MA—IC), Heart (MA—IC).

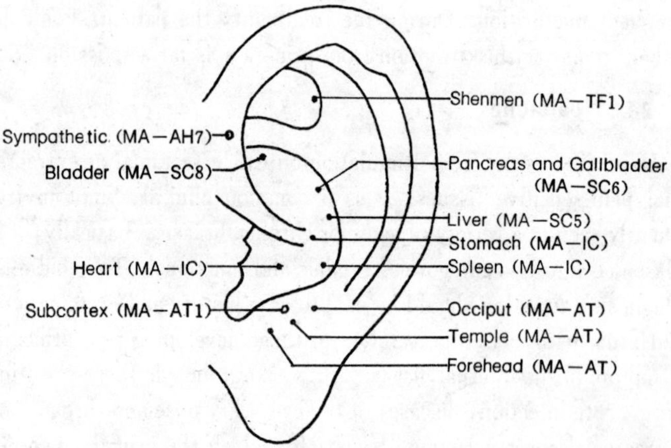

Fig. 5—24 Points for headache

Method: Apply auricular-point-pressing therapy with vaccaria seeds, magnetic beads or borneol. The opposite pressing or perpendicular pressing is recommended.

Basis for selection of points

The corresponding points to the diseased part are selected to promote the flow of Qi and Blood in the local region and dredge Channels to stop pain, that is, Forehead (MA—AT) for sincipital headache, Occiput (MA—AT) for the occipital headache, and Temple (MA—AT) for the temporal headache. Subcortex (Ma—AT1), Sympathetic (MA—AH7) and Shenmen (MA—TF1) are used to calm the mind and stop pain via regulating the cerebral cortex and autonomic vasomotoricity.

Add Stomach (MA—IC) to regulate the Yangming Channel for the sincipital headache, Gallbladder (MA—SC6) to dredge the Shaoyang Channel for the temporal headache, Gallbladder (MA—

SC8) to clear and regulate the Taiyang Channel for the occipital headache, and Liver (MA—SC5) to suppress the hyperactive Liver Yang and send down the adverse flow of Qi for the parietal headache. In case of the deficiency type of headache, Heart (MA—IC) and Spleen (MA—IC) are added to replenish the Heart and Spleen, to invigorate Qi and nourish Blood.

References for treatment

Li Hanjun reported 105 cases of headache treated with auricular-point-pressing therapy. Among them, 57 were nervous headache, 40 were vascular headache and the remaining 8 were typical migraine. The longest history of disease was 20 years and the shortest was 2 months. Main points used were: Shenmen (MA—TF1), Subcortex (MA—AT1), Occiput (MA—AT), Ear apex (MA—H6). Supplementary points were selected based on the Channel identification and syndrome identification according to the aching area of the head and accompanying symptoms. Vaccaria seeds were used to press the points once every 2—3 days with 7 treatment sessions constituting one course. After 2—15 treatment sessions, 59 cases were cured (54.2%), marked by complete pain relief without recurrence in half a year follow-up; 41 were improved, marked by evident pain relief with obvious decrease of recurrence; and 5 were ineffective. The total effective rate was 95.2%.

Wu Xiqiang reported 50 cases of headache treated by auricular-point- pressing therapy with *Bing Pian* (Borneolum Syntheticum). Main points selected were Shenmen (MA—TF1) and Subcortex (MA—AT1). Supplementary points were: Forehead (MA—AT) for sincipital headache, Temple (MA—AT), Liver (MA—SC5) and Gallbladder (MA—SC6) for temporal headache, Liver (MA—SC5) for parietal headache, and Occiput (MA—AT) and Bladder (MA—SC8) for occipital headache. Points were also selected according to syndrome identification, namely, Liver (MA—SC5) and Gallbladder (MA—SC6) for headache due to hyperactivity of the Liver Yang, Heart (MA—IC) and Spleen (MA—IC) for headache due to deficiency of Qi and Blood, and Lung (MA—IC1) and Spleen (MA—IC) for headache due to Phlegm-Turbidity. *Bing Pian* (Borneolum Syntheticum) of the size of 2—3 mm previously put on a piece of adhesive tape of 0.6×0.6 cm^2 was used to press the points. The treatment was carried out every 3 days. Result: cured in 34 cases (65%), marked by disappearance of pain and no recurrence within 3 months; remarkably improved in 10 cases (19.2%), marked by disappearance of pain, however, recurrence presented in 3 months; improved in 8 cases (15.4%), marked by reduced pain and frequency of the headache. The total effective rate was 100%.

Liu Xinlian reported 43 cases of migraine treated with auricular-point-pressing therapy at Shenmen (MA—TF1), Subcortex (MA—AT1), Heart (MA—IC), Liver (MA—SC5), Temple (MA—AT) and Endocrine (MA—IC3). Put the cross section of a half green gram that was previously cut into two equal parts on a piece of adhesive tape of 0.7×0.7 cm^2, and then tape it on a point for pressing. The Ear Apex (MA—H6) was pricked to cause bleeding. 5 treatment sessions constituted 1 therapeutic course. Result: cured in 18 cases (65%), marked by disappearance of pain and no recurrence in 3 months; improved in 24 cases (15.4%), marked by obvious pain relief and decrease of the frequency; and ineffective in 1 case. The total effective rate was 97.67%.

25. Postconcussional syndrome

Concussion of brain refers to transient dysfunction of the central nervous system immediately following a trauma of the head. After the patient regained consciousness, there may present such symptoms as retrograde amnesia, headache, dizziness, numbness in the head, nausea, tinnitus, lack of concentration, insomnia and dysfunction of the vegetative nerve. If the above symptoms last over 3 months, they are called postconcussional syndrome. Generally, examination on the nervous system finds no abnormality or just slight positive signs. Overwork, nervousness and insomnia may aggravate the above symptoms.

TCM holds that the head is the confluence of all the Yang Channels and the sea of Marrow. All the Essence of the Zang-Fu organs and lucid Yang Qi are transported to the head. Trauma of the head may cause stagnation of Qi and Blood leading to malnutrition of the brain. As a result, the above symptoms appear.

Point (Fig. 5—25) and method

Main points: Forehead (MA—AT), Occiput (MA—AT), Kidney (MA—SC), Subcortex (MA—AT1), Shenmen (MA—TF1), Central Rim (MA—AT).

Supplementary points: Heart (MA—IC), Sympathetic (MA—AH7), Stomach (MA—IC), Ear Apex (MA—H6).

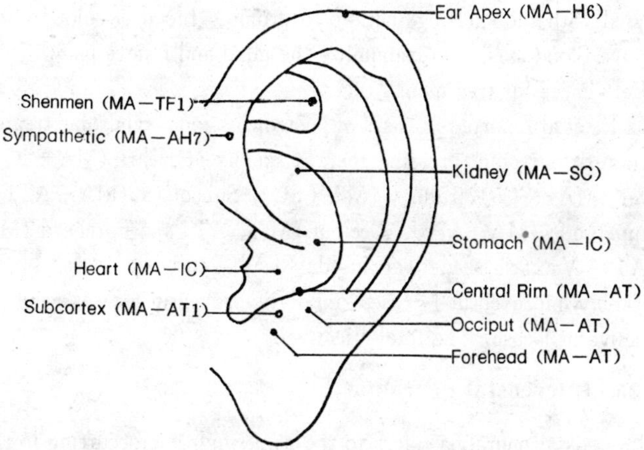

Fig. 5—25 Points for postconcussional syndrome

Method: Apply auricular-point-pressing with vaccaria seeds or magnetic beads. Plaster-sticking method with *Xiang Gui Huo Xue Gao* (Plaster for Promoting Blood Circulation with Moschus and Cortex Cinnamomi) or *Hou Xue Zhen Tong Gao* (Plaster for Promoting Blood Circulation to Relieve Pain) can also be employed. The perpendicular or opposite pressing approach is recommended.

Basis for selection of point

As the corresponding point to the aching area, Forehead (MA—AT) and Occiput (MA—AT) are selected to promote flow of Qi and Blood in the local Channels and Collaterals. Since the Kidney dominates the bones, generates Marrow and relates to the brain, Kidney (MA—SC) is selected in combination with Central Rim (MA—AT) to replenish the Kidney, to invigorate the brain and produce Marrow. Subcortex (MA—AT1) and Shenmen (MA—TF1) are used to tranquilize the mind and relieve pain. The joint use of the above points can activate Blood circulation, dredge Channels, replenish Essence, produce Marrow, calm the mind and stop pain.

For symptoms of vegetative nerve dysfunction, Sympathetic (MA—AH7) is added to regulate the vegetative nerve. For insomnia and poor memory, Heart (MA—IC) is added. For nausea and vomiting, Stomach (MA—IC) is added. For lingering illness, Ear Apex is treated with Bloodletting therapy to promote Blood circulation and remove Blood stasis, to tranquilize the mind and relieve pain.

References for treatment

Li Da et al reported 31 cases of postconcussional syndrome treated with auricular-point-pressing therapy mainly at Heart (MA—IC), Liver (MA—SC5), Kidney (MA—SC), Subcortex (MA—AT1), Sympathetic (MA—AH7), Occiput (MA—AT) and Forehead (MA—AT). Vaccaria seeds were used. Result: cured in 10 cases, remarkably improved in 14 cases, mildly improved in 6 cases, and ineffective in 1 case. The total effective rate was 96.8%.

26. Intercostal neuralgia

Intercostal neuralgia refers to the pain syndrome occurring in the supplied area of one or several intercostal nerves that are made up of the anterior branches of the spinal nerves from the second to the tenth thoracic nerves. Most of the disease are progressing and lingering and frequently encountered in youth and middle-aged women with anemia. Intercostal neuralgia is often seen as a symptom subsequent to other diseases such as pathological change or infection in the nearby tissues and organs, trauma, cold exposure, or herpes zoster which results in viral intercostal neuritis.

Intercostal neuralgia is manifested mainly by persistent pain with paroxysmal aggravation in one or several intercostal regions. The pain is usually stabbing or lancinating, involving the homolateral abdomen or shoulder and aggravated by breathing, cough and sneeze. Physical examination will find dermal hyperesthesia in the relevant intercostal region and tenderness on the costal margin.

In TCM, this disease belongs to the category of *Xie Tong* (Hypochondriac Pain). It is believed to be caused by emotional disturbance that brings about failure of the Liver in maintaining the normal flow of Qi, or sudden stumbling or twisting that injures the hypochondrium leading to stagnation of Qi and obstruction of Channels. Hypochondriac pain occurs subsequently.

Point (Fig. 5−26) and method

Main points: Chest (MA−AH11), Liver (MA−SC5), Pancreas and Gallbladder (MA−SC6), Shenmen (MA−TF1), Subcortex (MA−AT1), Endocrine (MA−IC3), Adrenal Gland (MA−T).

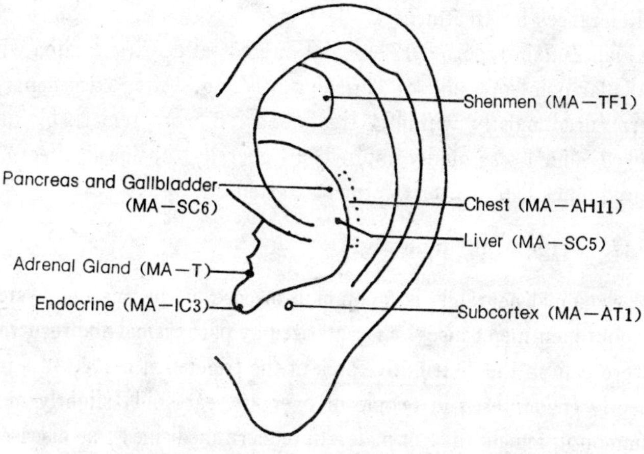

Fig. 5−26 Points for intercostal neuralgia

Method: Apply auricular-point-pressing therapy with vaccaria seeds. Plaster-sticking method can also be employed with *She Xiang Zhuang Gu Gao* (Plaster for Strengthening Bone Mainly with Moschus), *Huo Xue Zhi Tong Gao* (Plaster for Promoting Blood Circulation to Relieve Pain) or *Xiao Yan Zhi Tong Gao* (Plaster for Relieving Inflammation and Pain). The opposite pressing or perpendicular pressing with strong stimulation is recommended.

Basis for selection of point

This disease should be treated with primary therapeutic principle of promoting the circulation of Blood and dredging Channels to alleviate pain. As a corresponding point to the diseased area, Chest (MA – AH11) is selected to dredge local Channels and activate Blood circulation. Hypochondrium is the distributive area of the Liver Channel and Gallbladder Channel, Liver (MA – SC5) and Pancreas and Gallbladder (MA – SC6) are therefore combined with Chest (MA – AH11) to clear Channels and Collaterals, activate Blood and remove Blood stasis, promote the flow of Qi and relieve pain. Shenmen (MA – TF1) and Subcortex (MA – AT1) are two principal points for stopping pain. Endocrine (MA – IC3) and Adrenal Gland (MA – T) are supplemented to relieve inflammation and stop pain.

References for treatment

Guan Zunxin reported 12 cases of intercostal neuritis treated with auricular-point-pressing or auricular needling. After treatment, 8 were cured mostly within 4 treatments, 3 were remarkably improved, and 1 was mildly improved. Generally, analgesic effect appeared immediately after treatment started.

27. Trigeminal neuralgia

Trigeminal neuralgia is a common disease of the nervous system without identified causes, characterized by paroxysmal and recurrent severe pain in the distributive area of the trigeminal nerve. It is frequently encountered in people of over 40 years old, slightly more common in female than in male. In modern medicine, this disease is classified into primary type and secondary type. The etiology of the former is uncertain at present while the latter often occurs secondarily to cerebellopontile tumor, trigeminal ganglioma, angioma, arachnoiditis, etc. The application of auricular-sticking-pressing therapy is limited to the treatment of primary trigeminal neuralgia.

Trigeminal neuralgia manifests itself mainly by tearing, electrical, lancinating, stabbing or burning pain in the distributive area of the trigeminal nerve. Attacks are often induced by chewing, talking, brushing the teeth or washing the face, which may touch the trigger point. Each attack lasts several seconds or several minutes with a variable period of remission. A severe pain may be accompanied with reflex twitching of the facial muscle, lacrimation and conjunctival congestion. The pain is mostly unilateral, rarely bilateral. On objective examination, no positive signs can be found in primary trigeminal neuralgia while abnormal signs in the distributive area of the trigeminal nerve, such as retardation or disappearance of the corneal reflex, may be found in secondary one.

In TCM, trigeminal neuralgia belongs to the categories of *Mian Tong* (Facial Pain) and *Pian Tong Feng* (Migraine). It is considered to be caused by invasion of Wind-Cold or Wind-Heat, or ascending of excessive Heat from the Liver and Stomach leading to stagnation of Qi and Blood in the Channels and Collaterals of the face.

Point (Fig. 5—27) and method

Main points: Cheek (MA—L), Stomach (MA—IC), Liver (MA—SC5), Subcortex (MA—AT1), Shenmen (MA—TF1).

Supplementary points: Forehead (MA—AT), Jaw (MA—L), Ear Apex (MA—H6).

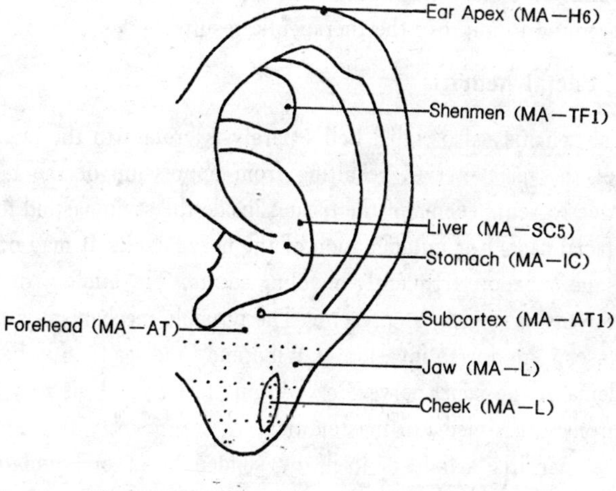

Fig. 5—27 Points for trigeminal neuralgia

Method: Apply auricular-point-pressing therapy with vaccaria seeds or magnetic beads. The opposite pressing or perpendicular pressing with strong stimulation is recommended.

Basis for selection of point

As a corresponding point to the diseased area, Cheek (MA—L) is selected to promote the flow of Qi and Blood in the facial Channels and Collaterals. Since the Stomach Channel passes through the face, Stomach (MA—IC) is used in combination with Liver (MA—SC5) to purge the excessive Fire of the Liver and the Stomach, clear Channels and Collaterals, promote the flow of Blood and relieve pain. Subcortex (MA—AT1) and Shenmen (MA—TF1) are two principal points for tranquilizing the mind and relieving pain. The joint use of the above points can achieve the purpose of purging the excessive Fire, dredging Channels and Collaterals, tranquilizing the mind and relieving pain. Add Forehead (MA—AT) for pain of the ocular branch, Jaw (MA—L) for pain of the maxillary branch, and Ear Apex (MA—H6), which is pricked to cause bleeding, for severe and lingering pain.

Remarks

Auricular-point-pressing therapy has proven quite effective for trigeminal neuralgia. In clinical practice, it is usually combined with body needling to improve the therapeutic results.

28. Facial neuritis

Facial neuritis, also called Bell's paralysis, refers to the impairment of the facial nerve, resulting from oppression of the facial nerve due to acute edema of the tissues inside the stylomastoid foramen (facial canal) or inflammation of the nerve itself. It may occur at any age but more frequently in young adults. The etiology of this disease remains unclear at present. The possible mechanism is that local vasospasm due to invasion of Wind and Cold leads to ischemia and edema of the facial nerve. In addition, facial paralysis may follow chronic otitis media or mastoiditis.

Facial neuritis manifests itself by sudden onset and unilateral mimetic paralysis marked by disappearance of frontal wrinkle, enlargement of palpebial fissure, flat nasolabial groove, ptosis of corner of the mouth, face drawn to the healthy side, inability of the affected side to frown, to raise the eyebrow, to close the eye, to show the teeth, to blow out the cheek and to pout the lips. When the patient has his meals, the food often retains in the buccal cavity of the affected side. In some patients, there may be hyperacusis or hypogeusia on the anterior 2/3 of the affected side of the tongue.

In TCM, facial neuritis belongs to the categories of *Mian Tan* (Facial Paralysis) and *Kou Yan Wo Xie* (Deviation of the Eye and Mouth). It is usually caused by invasion of Wind, Cold, Dampness or Heat into the Yangming Channel leading to malnutrition of the facial musculature.

Point (Fig. 5—28) and method

Main points: Cheek (MA—L), Mouth (MA—IC5), Eye (MA—L1), Liver (MA—SC5), Adrenal Gland (MA—T), Endocrine (MA—IC3).

Supplementary points: Ear Apex (MA—H6), Spleen (MA—IC), Subcortex (MA—AT1), Sympathetic (MA—AH7).

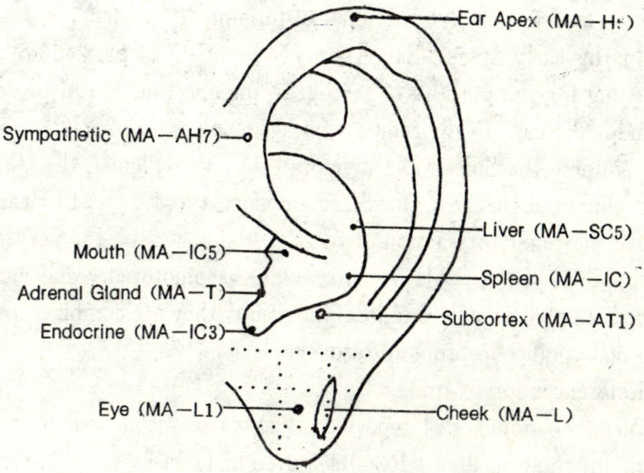

Fig. 5—28 Points for facial neuritis

Method: Apply auricular-point-pressing therapy with vaccaria seeds. Plaster-sticking therapy can also be employed with *Xiang Gui Hou Xue Gao* (Plaster for Promoting Blood Circulation Mainly with Moschus and Cortex Cinnamomi) or *Xiao Yan Zhi Tong Gao*

(Plaster for Relieving Inflammation and Pain). The opposite pressing or perpendicular pressing with strong stimulation is recommended. In the early stage, Bloodletting at Ear Apex (MA−H6) may be used.

Basis for selection of point

This disease should be treated with the therapeutic principle of dispelling Wind, activating Blood and dredging Channels. Cheek (MA−L), Mouth (MA−IC5) and Eye (MA−L1) are selected as the corresponding point to the diseased area to dispel Wind detained in the face, to clear the facial Channels and regulate flow of Qi and Blood. TCM holds that all Wind syndromes, tremors and vertigo are mainly due to the dysfunction of the Liver, for the Liver governs the smooth flow of Qi and is attributed to wood according the theory of Five Elements. Therefore, Liver (MA−SC5) is used to soothe the movement of Qi, to relieve the depressed Liver and to calm the pathological Wind. Adrenal Gland (MA−AT) and Endocrine (MA−IC3) have anti-inflammatory and antirheumatic efficacy, so they are selected to promote the relief of inflammatory edema.

In the early stage, Ear Apex (MA − H6) is pricked to cause bleeding for the purpose of strengthening the function of dispelling Wind and Heat. In the remission stage, Spleen (MA−IC) is added to reinforce the Spleen and invigorate Qi, to replenish the Vital Qi and eliminate the Evil Qi. Since Subcortex (MA − AT1) can improve the regulatory action of the cerebral cortex on the nerves and Sympathetic (MA − AH7) can regulate vasomotoricity and increase Blood supply to ameliorate local nutrition, they are combined to help the main points to promote recovery.

References for treatment

Yang Zhaomin et al reported 24 cases of facial neuritis treated with auricular needling. Results: cured in 12 cases (57%), remarkably improved in 9 cases (29%), mildly improved in 2 cases (9%), and ineffective in 1 case. The total effective rate was 95%. In a control group (n = 25) treated with body needling, cured in 18 cases (72%), remarkably improved in 3 cases (12%), mildly improved in 2 cases (8%), and ineffective in 2 cases. The total effective rate was 92%. Statistic analysis of the effects showed no significant difference between the two groups.

Zhen Lianfu reported 136 cases of facial paralysis treated with needle-embedding therapy mainly at Liver (MA – SC5), Spleen (MA – IC), Subcortex (MA – AT1), Shenmen (MA – TF1), Cheek (MA – L) and Forehead (MA – AT). 4 – 5 of the above points in the affected side were used in each treatment with one therapeutic course lasting one week. Result: cured in 97 cases (71.32%), remarkably improved in 19 cases (13.97%), mildly improved in 15 cases (11.03%), and ineffective in 1 case (0.75). Because 4 patients discontinued the treatment, they were not included. The total effective rate was 96.32%.

Ji Jiangge reported 160 cases of facial paralysis treated with auricular Bloodletting therapy. On the posterior surface of the auricle of the affected side, select an obvious blood vessel near the helix. First knead it for several minutes to cause congestion, then sterilize that area. Stabilize the auricle with the left thumb and middle finger and hold a small surgical knife blade with the right hand, cut the selected vessel to bleed 2—3 ml, afterwards clear away the bloodstain and cover the wound with sterilized dressing. During the following week, ask the patient to avoid wetting the wound for fear of infection. For mild cases with a short duration, the disease can be cured after only one treatment, while for severe cases with a long duration, 2—4 treatments performed once per week and alternate use of two vessels may be required. Result: cured in 154 cases and ineffective in 6 cases. The cure rate was 95%.

Remarks

Auricular-point-pressing therapy is suitable for facial neuritis in the progressive stage. When the disease is in the remission period, body needling can be combined to improve therapeutic effects and shorten treatment period.

29. Facial spasm

Facial spasm refers to the paroxysmal irregular muscular spasm on one side of the face. Its etiology remains unclear and is possibly associated with pathological stimulation on the facial nerve. A few develop from facial neuritis. This disease mostly occurs in the middle-aged and elderly people, especially in female.

Facial spasm manifests itself by spasm mostly beginning from the intermittent slight spasm of the orbicularis oculi and progressing to other facial muscles on the same side. The spasm of the mouth corner is the most obvious. Spasm may be aggravated by mental stress, fatigue, active physical movement and concentration on the focus, but relieved completely during the sleep. In general, no pain is felt by the patient and no positive signs are found in examination on the nervous system.

As a chronic and progressive disease, facial spasm cannot be relieved spontaneously. Some cases may develop into complete facial paralysis several years later. In Western medicine, there is no effective therapy at present.

In TCM, facial spasm belongs to the categories of *Jin Ti Rou Shun* (Muscular Twitching and Cramp), *Yan Mian Chou Chu* (Facial Tic) and *Yan Jian Shun Dong* (Twitching of Eyelid).

Point (Fig. 5−29) and method

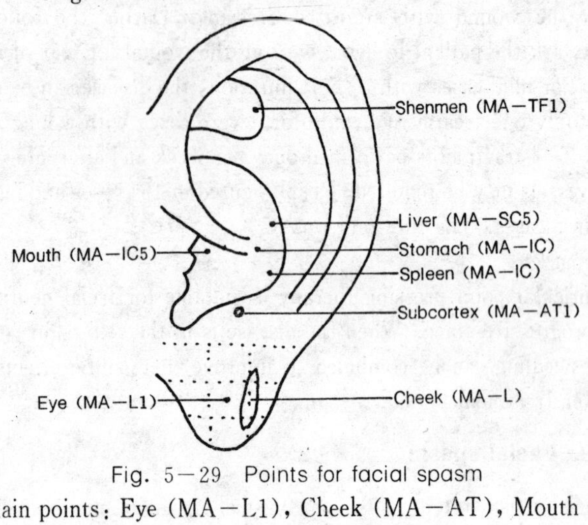

Fig. 5−29 Points for facial spasm

Main points: Eye (MA−L1), Cheek (MA−AT), Mouth (MA−IC5), Stomach (MA−IC), Liver (MA−SC5), Spleen (MA−

IC).

Supplementary points: Subcortex (MA－AT1), Shenmen (MA－TF1).

Method: Apply auricular-point-pressing therapy with vaccaria seeds or magnetic beads. The opposite pressing or perpendicular pressing is recommended.

Basis for selection of point

As the points corresponding to the diseased area, Eye (MA－L1), Cheek (MA－AT) and Mouth (MA－IC5) are selected to dispel Wind and relax the muscles and tendons. Since the Stomach Channel passes through the face, the Spleen dominates the muscles and serves as the acquired constitution, and the Liver is in charge of the tendons, Stomach (MA－IC), Spleen (MA－IC) and Liver (MA－SC5) are used to clear and activate Channels and Collaterals, enrich Blood and nourish tendons, to calm Wind and relieve spasm. Subcortex (MA－AT1) and Shenmen (MA－TF1) can regulate the cerebral cortex and tranquilize the mind, so they are selected to strengthen the function of calming the mind and relieving spasm.

References for treatment

Wei Hongping reported 7 cases of intractable facial spasm treated with auricular-point-pressing therapy, of which the longest case history was 4 years while the shortest 10 months. All of the patients had previously tried herbal medicine, Western medicine or physiotherapy but received little effects. Points selected were: Cheek (MA－AT), Eye (MA－L1), Mouth (MA－IC5), Shenmen (MA－TF1), Liver (MA－SC5), Spleen (MA－IC), Occiput (MA－AT), Subcortex (MA－AT1). Treatment with vaccaria seeds was carried out once per week with 5 treatments constituting 1 course. Result: cured in 4 cases, marked by disappearance of spasm; remarkably improved in 3 cases, marked by obvious relief of spasm which may reappear when the patient was in fatigue or overstress. The shortest course of treatment was 4 weeks while the longest 10 weeks.

Wang Yi reported 34 cases of blepharospasm treated with auricular -point-pressing therapy, of which the shortest case history was 1 month while the longest 3 months. Points selected were: Liver (MA−SC5), Shenmen (MA−TF1), Subcortex (MA−AT1) and Eye (MA−L1) as the main points, and Spleen (MA−IC) and Occiput (MA−AT) as the supplementary points. Vaccaria seeds were used in treatment and the stuck seeds were changed once every 3 days with 5 times constituting one therapeutic course. After one course of treatment, pafients weve cured in 26 cases (75.5%), marked by disappearance of symptoms, and remarkably improved in 8 cases (23.5%), marked by obvious relief of symptoms. The total effective rate was 100%.

Remarks

Auricular-point-pressing therapy presents satisfactory short-term effects for facial spasm and has advantages over body needling which, by treating facial points directly, can cause overexcitation of local nerves and aggravate spasm of local muscles.

30. Cerebrovascular accident

Cerebrovascular accident results from acute disturbance of cerebral circulation which leads to acute or subacute cerebral impairment, characterized by sudden disorder of consciousness, aphasia, paralysis, etc. It can be classified into two categories: the hemorrhagic and the ischemic. The former includes cerebral hemorrhage and subarachnoid hemorrhage, while the latter comprises cerebral thrombosis and cerebral embolism.

After acute stage (2 weeks to 1 month), the following symptoms may be left such as complete or incomplete unilateral paralysis, weakness, anesthesia, central facial paralysis, dysphasia, dysphagia, etc. If the disease lasts within half a year, it is considered to develep into the remission stage, while if over half a year, into the sequel stage.

In TCM, cerebrovascular accident belongs to the category of *Zhong Feng* (Windstroke).

Point (Fig. 5−30) and method

Main points: Points corresponding to the paralyzed parts, Subcortex (MA−AT1), Liver (MA−SC5), Spleen (MA−IC).

Supplementary points: Heart (MA－IC), Tongue (MA－L), Sympathetic (MA－AH7), Esophagus (MA－IC6), Pharynx and Larynx (MA－T3), Mouth (MA－IC5), Cheek (MA－L).

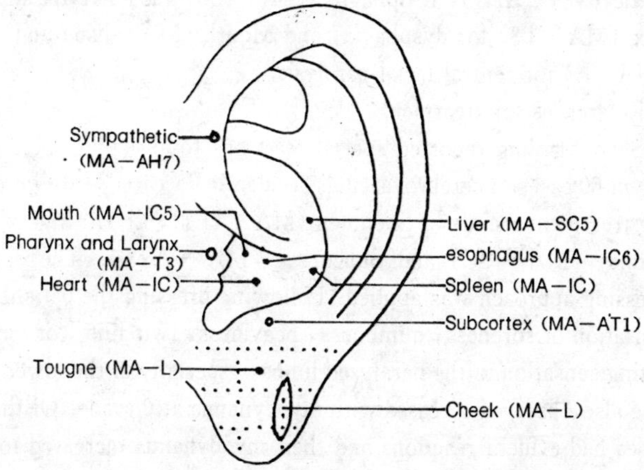

Fig. 5－30 Points for cerebrovascular accident

Method: Apply auricular-point-pressing therapy with vaccaria seeds. Plaster-sticking therapy with *Xiang Gui Hou Xue Gao* (Plaster for Promoting Blood Circulation Mainly with Moschus and Cortex Cinnamomi) can also be used. The opposite pressing, perpendicular pressing or intermittent pressing can be selected according to pathological conditions.

Basis for selection of point

According to the paralyzed limbs, the corresponding points are selected to dredge Channels and Collaterals and regulate Qi and Blood in the affected area. For example, Hip (MA－AH4), Knee (MA－AH3) and Ankle (MA－AH2) are selected for paralysis of the leg. Subcortex (MA－AT1) is used to regulate the cerebral cortical function and promote the movement of limbs. The Spleen dominates the limb muscle, the Liver stores Blood and controls tendons and the Stomach connects with Yangming Channel which is rich in Qi and Blood. Therefore, Spleen (MA－IC), Stomach (MA－IC) and Liver (MA－SC5) are selected to strengthen the Spleen and invigorate Qi, enrich Blood and nourish the Liver, activate Blood and relax tendons, which are beneficial to the recovery of limb movement. Add Heart (MA—IC) and Tongue (MA—L) for dysphasia, Sympathetic (MA—AH7), Esophagus (MA—IC6) and Pharynx and Larynx (MA—T3) for dysphagia, and Mouth (MA—IC5) and Cheek (MA—L) for central facial paralysis.

References for treatment

Shao Xiaoling reported special reactions to auricular-point-pressing in 60 cases of cerebrovascular accident. Vaccaria seeds were used for treatment mainly at Shenmen (MA—TF1), Liver (MA—SC5), Kidney (MA—SC) and Subcortex (MA—AT1). The opposite pressing approach was applied. Following pressing the patient felt a sensation of soreness, numbness, heaviness, twitching, or upwards lifting sensation in the paralyzed limbs, especially in the lower limb. She also observed 13 cases with myodynamia at 0 grade. Of them, 9 cases had evident reactions and their myodynamia increased to 3—4 grade after 1—3 treatment courses. The author of this article believed that those sensitive to this therapy would obtain quicker improvement than those insensitive, which had reference value for prognosis.

Cao Suoqi et al reported a trial in which the alteration of the cerebrovascular function upon auricular-point-pressing therapy was observed in 53 healthy subjects. Result revealed that in EEG the amplitude of wave was raised, the ascending angle was enlarged, and the rate of dicrotic wave was increased after auricular-point-pressing with vaccaria seeds at Heart (MA—IC), Subcortex (MA—AT1) and Forehead (MA—AT). Statistic analysis showed significant difference before and after treatment ($P<0.05$).

Remarks

Auricular-point-pressing therapy is suitable for cerebrovascular accident in the restoration stage, and also effective for that in the sequel stage. The effect of the latter, however, is not as good as the former.

During the treatment, the patient should be encouraged to do functional training. When Shoulder (MA—SF4), Elbow (MA—

SF3), Hip (MA－AH4) or Knee (MA－AH3) is being pressed, the patient may feel a sensation of hot or twitch in the corresponding area. At that moment, ask the patient to raise his paralyzed limbs as far as possible. Usually, an instant increase of myodynamia will appear. This procedure should be performed several times daily, which can promote the recovery.

31. Neurosism

Neurosism is a common nervous disease with a slow onset and a protracted course, frequently encountered in young adults. It is largely induced by psychic trauma, long-term mental overwork, tension or fatigue, which causes imbalance between cortical excitation and inhibition and a considerable number of symptoms involving mutisystem. The main mental symptoms include insomnia, dream-disturbed sleep, irritability, anxiety, unreasonably suspicion, lassitude and poor memory. They may be accompanied with symptoms due to dysfunction of the vegetative nerve, such as palpitation, profuse sweating, cold or numb limbs, decrease of sexual desire and irregular menstruation. No organic change is found.

In TCM, neurosism belongs to the categories of *Bu Mei* (Insomnia) and *Yu Zheng* (Depression Syndrome). It is considered to be caused by emotional impairment or general weakness due to a severe or lingering disease causing dysfunction of the Zang-Fu organs.

Point (Fig. 5－31) and method

Main points: Heart (MA－IC), Kidney (MA－SC), Shenmen (MA－TF1), Subcortex (MA－AT1), Central Rim (MA－AT), Anterior Ear Lobe (MA－L).

Supplementary points: Spleen (MA－IC), Stomach (MA－IC), Liver (MA－SC5), Pancreas and Gallbladder (MA－SC6).

Method: Apply auricular-point-pressing therapy with vaccaria seeds or magnetic beads. The perpendicular pressing or intermittent pressing is recommended. For mild cases in the early stage, finger pressing or massage is recommended.

Basis for selection of point

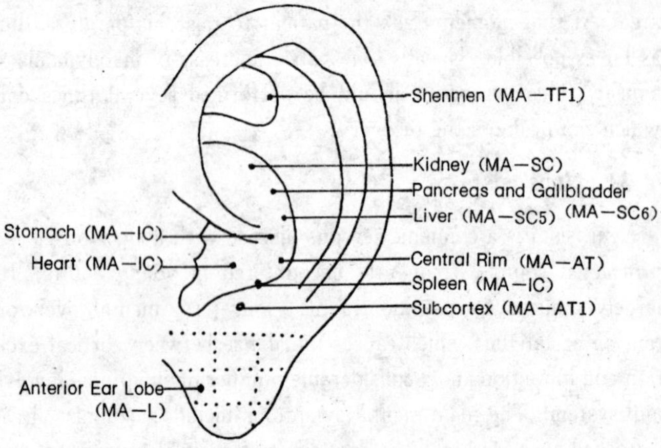

Fig. 5—31 Points for neurosism

This disease should be treated with the principle of calming the mind and regulating Zang-Fu organs. Heart (MA—IC) is selected to relieve mental stress and calm the mind. Kidney (MA—SC) is used to invigorate the brain and replenish the Kidney which, according to TCM theory, stores Essence and generates Marrow. Shenmen (MA—TF1), Subcortex (MA—AT1) and Central Rim (MA—AT) are combined with the above points to regulate the cerebral cortical function and restore its excito-inhibitory balance. Anterior Ear Lobe (MA—L), as an empirical point for neurosism, functions to calm the mind and induce sleep. According to the accompanying symptoms, Spleen (MA—IC), Stomach (MA—IC), Liver (MA—SC5) or/and Gallbladder (MA—SC6) are added to regulate and harmonize the functions of Zang-Fu organs and improve the efficacy of tranquilizing and calming the mind, invigorating the brain and benefiting sleep.

References for treatment

Huang Lichun reported 166 cases of neurosism treated with auricular -point-pressing therapy mainly at Ear Apex (MA—H6), Shenmen (MA—TF1), Heart (MA—IC), Occiput (MA—AT) and Subcortex (MA—AT1). Supplementary points were added on the basis of TCM syndrome identification. Green grams were used for treatment and they were changed once every 3—5 days with 6 treatment sessions constituting one course. Result: cured in 60 cases (36.1%), marked by more than 6 hours' sleep each night without hypnotic; remarkably improved in 39 cases (23.5%), marked by more than 6 hours' sleep each night without hypnotic, ameliorated symptoms, but recurrence after the treatment was discontinued; mildly improved in 43 cases (25.9%), marked by obvious improvement of the sleep (quick to fall asleep and able to fall asleep again if waking up, the sleeping time increased by 2—3 hours each night) and that of subjective symptoms; and ineffective in 24 cases (14.5%). The total effective rate was 85.5%.

Gao Zhenzi reported 150 cases of neurosism treated with auricular- point-pressing therapy. Points selected were: Shenmen (MA—TF1), Heart (MA—IC), Spleen (MA—IC) and Subcortex (MA—AT1) as main points, Lung (MA—IC1), Kidney (MA—SC), Small Intestine (MA—SC2), Occiput (MA—AT) and Forehead (MA—AT) as supplementary points. Green grams were used for treatment and the seeds were changed once every other day with 10 treatment sessions constituting one course. Result: remarkably improved in 108 cases, marked by disappearance of symptoms and 6—8 hours' sleep each night after one week treatment; mildly improved in 34 cases, marked by obviously ameliorated symptoms and 5 hours' sleep each night; and ineffective in 8 cases. The total effective rate was 94.7%.

Jin Yaping reported 47 cases of neurosism treated with auricular-point-pressing therapy. Points selected were: Shenmen (MA—TF1), Heart (MA—IC), Subcortex (MA—AT1) and Occiput (MA—AT) as main points, Liver (MA—SC5), Spleen (MA—IC), Stomach (MA—IC) and Kidney (MA—SC) as supplementary points. *Xiang Gui Huo Xue Gao* (Plaster for Promoting Blood Circulation with Moschus and Cortex Cinnamomi) and green grams were used for treatment and they were changed every 3 days with 10 treatment sessions constituting one course. Result: cured in 7 cases, marked by disappearance of symptoms; remarkably improved in 22 cases, marked by obviously ameliorated symptoms; mildly improved in 18 cases, marked by ameliorated symptoms which, however, are not stable.

32. Hysteria

Hysteria is a common kind of psychoneurosis, frequently occurring in young people, especially in women. Obvious psychic trauma often serves as an induction factor of onset. It has the characteristics of repeated attacks and similar symptoms. Although the symptoms are complicated, they are manifested mainly by disturbances of the psyche, movement and sensation, possibly accompanied with dysfunction of the viscera and vegetative nerve. Mental symptoms include abnormal cry and laugh, shouting and making big trouble, dancing with joy, even dramatic performance or temporal stuporous state, etc. Common motion symptoms include aphasia, paralysis, tremor and spasm of limbs. Sensory symptoms include sudden loss of vision or blindness, deafness, foreign body sensation in the throat, vomiting and hiccup due to dysfunction of the vegetative nerve. However, careful physical examination fails to find positive signs in accordance with the symptoms.

In TCM, hysteria belongs to the categories of *Zang Zao* (Dry Zang Organs), *Jue Zheng* (*Syncope*), Yu Zheng (Depression Syndrome) and *Mei He Qi* (Globus Hystericus).

Point (Fig. 5—32) and method

Main points: Heart (MA—IC), Liver (MA—SC5), Shenmen (MA—TF1), Subcortex (MA—AT1), Central Rim (MA—AT).

Supplementary points: Points corresponding to diseased area.

Method: Apply auricular-point-pressing therapy with vaccaria seeds or magnetic beads. The opposite pressing or perpendicular pressing with strong stimulation is recommended.

Basis for selection of point

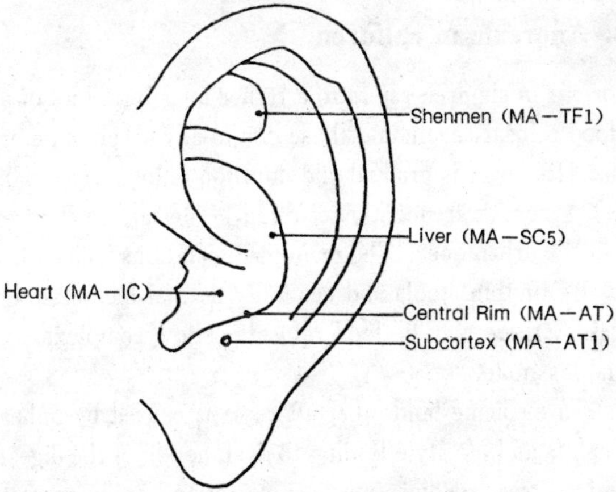

Fig. 5—32 Points for hysteria

This disease should be treated with the principle of tranquilizing and calming the mind, soothing the Liver and regulating Qi movement. Heart (MA—IC), Liver (MA—SC5), Shenmen (MA—TF1), Subcortex (MA—AT1) and Central Rim (MA—AT) are selected to regulate cerebral cortical function, to tranquilize and calm the mind. In case of exciting mental symptoms such as abnormal cry and laugh, or motion symptoms such as tremor and spasm of limbs, Occiput (MA—AT) and Forehead (MA—AT) are added to improve the efficacy of tranquilizing. In case of paralysis of the limb or stupor, points corresponding to the affected parts are added. In case of hysterical amaurosis or blindness, Eye (MA—L1), Eye1 (MA—L) and Eye2 (MA—L) are added. In case of deafness, Internal Ear (MA—L) is added. In case of foreign body sensation in the throat, Pharynx and Larynx (MA—T3) is added. In case of aphasia, Tongue (MA—L), Mouth (MA—IC5) and Pharynx and Larynx (MA—T3) are added. In case of vomiting and hiccup, Esophagus (MA—IC6) and Stomach (MA—IC) are added.

Remarks

Auricular-point-pressing therapy has proven quite effective for hysteria. However, because it is a psychic disease, combined use of suggestion therapy may produce dramatic results.

33. Anorexia in children

Anorexia in children refers to a rather long-term loss of appetite, even food refusal, excluding those due to any other acute or chronic diseases. Its onset is gradual and duration is long (generally over 1 month). Anorexia frequently occurs in 1—6 year-old children, especially in the urban ones. The main manifestations include loss of appetite, dry or thin stools and generally normal mental state. In severe cases, there may be food refusal, sallow complexion, emaciation and lassitude.

Western medicine holds that anorexia is caused by unhealthy dietetic habits and life style leading to dysfunction of the digestive system and decrease of digestive juice secretion, or by mental factors reducing the excitability of the food center, or by lack of trace elements bringing about hypogeusesthesia.

In TCM, it belongs to the categories of *Wu Shi* (Aversion to Food), *Shang Shi* (Damage of Improper Diet) and *Shi Zhi* (Retention of Food). TCM holds that anorexia in children is mainly due to deficiency of the Spleen and Stomach which fails in receiving food, transforming and transporting Food Essence.

Point (Fig. 5—33) and method

Main points: Stomach (MA—IC), Spleen (MA—IC), Small Intestine (MA—SC2), Pancreas and Gallbladder (MA—SC6).

Supplementary points: Subcortex (MA — AT1), Sympathetic (MA—AH7), Large Intestine (MA—SC4), Sanjiao (MA—IC4).

Method: Apply auricular-point-pressing therapy with vaccaria seeds. The intermittent pressing is recommended. Finger-pressing can be performed daily by the patient himself.

Basis for selection of point

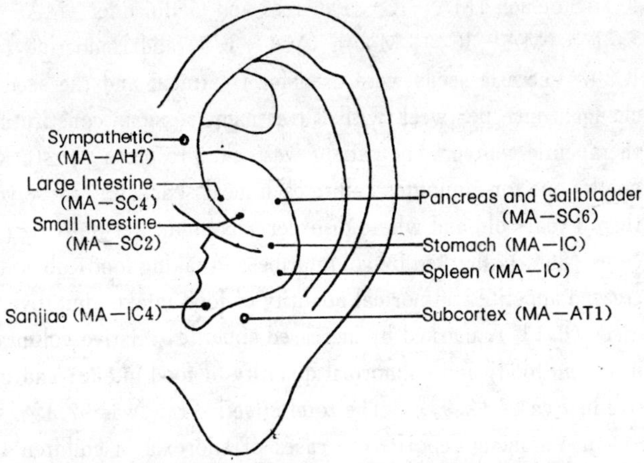

Fig. 5—33 Points for anorexia syndrome in children

This disease should be treated with the therapeutic principle of invigorating the Spleen and Stomach. Stomach (MA—IC) and Spleen (MA—IC) are selected to replenish the above two organs to facilitate transformation and transportation of Food Essence. Small Intestine (MA—SC2) and Pancreas and Gallbladder (MA—SC6) are selected to regulate digestive and absorptive functions of the intestinal tract and increase secretion of digestive juice which is helpful to induce appetite. For those resulting from emotional factors, Subcortex (MA—AT1) and Sympathetic (MA—AH7) are added to regulate the cerebral cortical function and increase the excitability of the appetite center. In case of stools being sometimes dry and sometimes thin, Large Intestine (MA—SC4) and Sanjiao (MA—IC4) are added to regulate the Intestine. The joint use of the above points can reach the purpose of strengthening the Spleen and Stomach to increase appetite.

References for treatment

Hou Rui reported 356 cases of anorexia in children treated with auricular-point-pressing, of which the shortest disease duration was 5 days while the longest 14 days, and the eldest was 9 years while the youngest 2 months. Main points selected were Spleen (MA—

IC), Stomach (MA—IC), Pancreas and Gallbladder (MA—SC6), Sanjiao (MA—IC4), Mouth (MA—IC5) and Endocrine (MA—IC3). Vaccaria seeds were used for treatment and the seeds were changed once per week with 3 treatment sessions constituting one therapeutic course. The patient was asked to press the stuck seeds one by one for 5 minutes before each meal, excluding those younger than 6 years old and whose disorder was mild. Result: cured in 210 cases (89%), marked by voluntariness in taking food, obviously increased appetite and normal quantity of food intake; improved in 19 cases (8.1%), marked by increased appetite, relative voluntariness in taking food, and subnormal quantity of food intake; and ineffective in 7 cases (2.9%). The total effective rate was 97.1%.

Cui Yunmeng reported 40 cases of anorexia in children treated with auricular-point-pressing therapy. Vaccaria seeds were used in this treatment. Result: remarkably effective in 32 cases (80%), and effective in 8 cases (20%). The total effective rate was 100%. Comparing the effect with that in a control group treated with medicine, there was a significant difference ($P<0.05$) in favor of the auricular therapy.

Wei Ling reported 100 cases of anorexia in children treated with auricular-point-pressing therapy, of which the shortest disease duration was 3 weeks while the longest 2 years. The points selected were Spleen (MA—IC), Stomach (MA—IC), Liver (MA—SC5), Small Intestine (MA—SC2), Heart (MA—IC) and Sympathetic (MA—AH7). Vaccaria seeds were used for treatment and they were changed every other day with alternate use of the two ears. Ten treatment sessions constituted one therapeutic course. After 2 courses of treatment, 39 cases got an obvious increase of food intake (food increased by 50—100g in each meal), 48 cases got a mild increase of food intake (food increased by 25—50g in each meal), and 13 cases had no response. The total effective rate was 87%. A follow-up of 40 cases conducted 2 months after the treatment was discontinued showed that the effects remained stable.

34. Restlessness syndrome in children

Restlessness syndrome in children, also called mild brain dysfunction (MBD), is a common behavior disorder syndrome, mostly occurring in preschool children. Its etiology remains unknown and is generally believed to be associated with heredity, mild injury of brain tissue, metabolic abnormalities of intracranial neurotransmitter, or motion instead of language to express psychological activities.

Children suffering from this disorder have normal or approximately normal intelligence. This is a comprehensive disease resulting from a variety of factors. It manifests itself by hyperactivity that is not in conformity with the child's intelligence, lack of concentration, unstable emotion, emotional impulse, various degrees of difficulty in study, and mild disturbance of the central nervous system such as dysfunction of perception, speech, memory, formation of conception and motion control. Lack of concentration and restlessness are the main characteristics. Research has revealed that about half of the victims show slight or moderate abnormal ECG, suggesting deficiency of the cerebral cortical waking action.

In TCM, there is no corresponding term to the disease. According to the manifestations, it may be classified into the categories of *Shen Qi Shi Chang* (Mental Disarrangement), *Feng Zheng* (Wind Syndrome) and *Fan Zao* (Restlessness).

Point (Fig. 5—34) and method

Main points: Kidney (MA—SC), Heart (MA—IC), Subcortex (MA—AT1), Central Rim (MA—AT).

Supplementary points: Liver (MA—SC5), Shenmen (MA—TF1), Spleen (MA—IC), Excitation Point (MA).

Method: Apply auricular-point-pressing therapy with vaccaria seeds. The intermittent pressing is recommended. Finger-pressing at the above points is also applicable.

Basis for selection of point

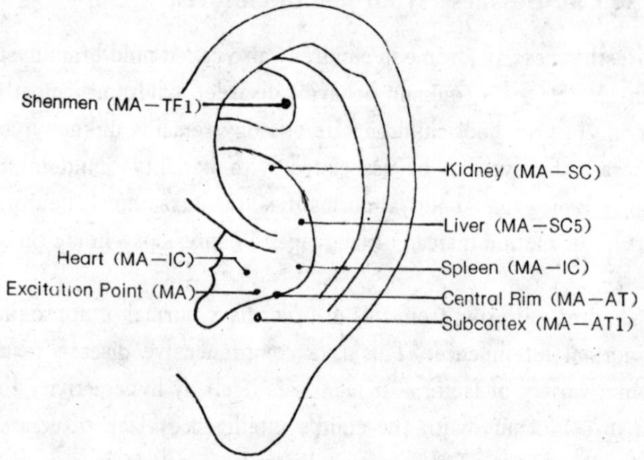

Fig. 5—34 Points for restlessness syndrome in children

TCM holds that this disease is caused by deficiency of the Heart and Kidney and imbalance of Yin and Yang leading to disturbance of mental activity. Therefore, treatment should be based on the therapeutic principle of replenishing the Kidney Essence, tonifying the Heart and tranquilizing the mind. Since the Kidney stores Essence that generates Marrow, the brain serves as the sea of the Marrow, and the Heart controls mental activities, Kidney (MA—SC) and Heart (MA—IC) are selected to replenish the Kidney Essence, enrich the Blood, calm the mind, and reinforce the brain Marrow. Subcortex (MA—AT1) and Central Rim (MA—AT) are used to regulate the excito-inhibitory function of the cerebral cortex and also to nourish the brain and calm the mind, which are beneficial to concentration of mind. In case of emotional instability and irritability, Liver (MA—SC5) and Shenmen (MA—TF1) are added to tranquilize and calm the mind, suppress the hyperactive Liver to stop Wind. For cases with poor appetite, Spleen (MA—IC) is added to invigorate the Spleen and the Stomach. If abnormalities are found in ECG, Excitation Point (MA) is added to improve the action of the cortical waking center.

References for treatment

Yun Shiyu et al reported 64 cases of mild brain dysfunction (MBD) treated with auricular-point-pressing therapy mainly at Kidney (MA－SC), Subcortex (MA－AT1) and Excitation Point (MA). Supplementary points were added: Liver (MA－SC5) for irritability, Heart (MA－IC) for poor memory and dream-disturbed sleep, and Spleen (MA－IC) for poor appetite. Vaccaria seeds were used in the treatment and the seeds were changed twice per week with alternate use of the two ears. Fifteen treatments constituted one therapeutic course. After half a year treatment, 51 cases were improved, marked by ameliorated symptoms that were close to normal, raised school record. The total effective rate was 79.7%. In a control group (n=30) without any treatment, only 4 cases obtained improvement (13.3%) after half a year's observation. Statistic analysis showed a significant difference between the effects of the two groups in favor of the treatment ($P<0.001$). Among the 26 cases with abnormal ECG in the treatment group, after half a year treatment, ECG returned to normal in 10 cases, improved in 9 cases and did not change in 6 cases. The improvement rate of ECG was 76%, significantly different from that before treatment ($P<0.01$).

Remarks

Auricular-point-pressing is effective for MBD. However, improvement or recovery needs a rather long-term treatment. Therefore, encourage the child or his/her relatives to persist in treatment. After obvious improvement has obtained, instruct the child or his/her relatives to help the child perform self-treatment with finger pressing approach, which is useful to stabilize the effectiveness.

At present, there are various medicines for MBD. However, disadvantages such as long-term treatment course and side-effects present to be a problem. Although auricular therapy needs a long-term treatment, the effects obtained are stable, the performance is easy, and side-effects are absent. Therefore, it is easily accepted by children and worthy to be spreaded.

Ⅱ. Orthopedic and Surgical Diseases

1. Stiffneck

Stiffneck refers to simple acute rigidity and pain with difficulty in the movement of the neck. It is mostly caused by long-term stretch of cervical muscle due to improper posture of the head during the sleep, or by invasion of Wind-Cold into the cervical muscle.

Stiffneck manifests itself mainly by stiffness or wryness of the neck with difficulty in turning left and right or bending forwards and extending backwards, which presents after getting up. Soreness and pain occur on the affected side of the neck and may radiate to the ipsilateral shoulder and arm. Physical examination finds spasm and tenderness of the local muscle without reddening or swelling.

In Western medicine, such diseases as cervicomuscular strain, sprain and contusion of the neck and retrograde degeneration of the cervical vertebrae can be refereed to as stiffneck for treatment.

Point (Fig. 5—35) and method

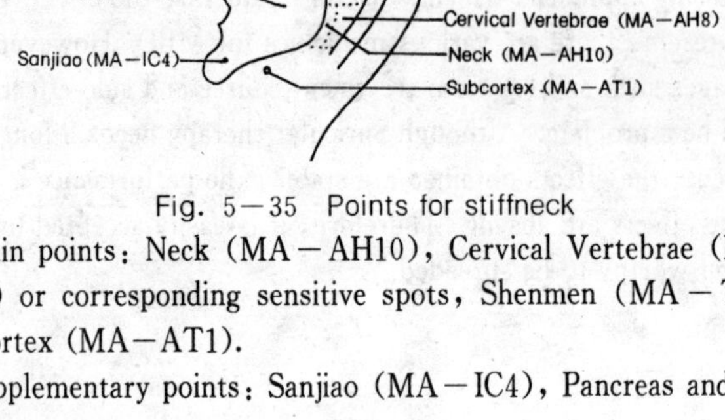

Fig. 5—35 Points for stiffneck

Main points: Neck (MA—AH10), Cervical Vertebrae (MA—AH8) or corresponding sensitive spots, Shenmen (MA—TF1), Subcortex (MA—AT1).

Supplementary points: Sanjiao (MA—IC4), Pancreas and Gallbladder (MA－SC6), Bladder (MA－SC8), Small Intestine (MA－SC2).

Method: Apply auricular-point-pressing therapy with vaccaria seeds. Plaster-sticking approach with *Shang Shi Zhi Tong Gao* (Plaster for Dispelling Dampness and Relieving Pain) or *Huo Xue Zhi Tong Gao* (Plaster for Promoting Blood Circulation to Relieve Pain) is also applicable. The opposite pressing or perpendicular pressing is recommended.

Basis for selection of point

Neck (MA－AH10), Cervical vertebrae (MA－AH8) or corresponding sensitive spots are selected to promote the flow of Qi and Blood, relax tendons and dredge Collaterals. Shenmen (MA－TF1) and Subcortex (MA－AT1) are two principal points for tranquilizing the mind and relieving pain. Combined use of the above points can reach the purpose of dredging Channels and Collaterals, activating Blood flow and stopping pain. For the Shaoyang type characterized by pain and evident limitation of neck movement to the left and right, Gallbladder (MA－SC6) and Sanjiao (MA－IC4) are added. For the Taiyang type characterized by pain and evident limitation of neck movement forewords and backwards, Bladder (MA－SC8) and Small Intestine (MA－SC2) are added.

References for treatment

Ma Yong reported 40 cases of stiffneck treated with auricular-point- pressing at Neck (MA－AH10), Occiput (MA－AT), Shenmen (MA－TF1), Adrenal Gland (MA－T) and External Genitals (MA－H4). Vaccaria seeds, which previously processed with Fructus Foenicuii and Rhizoma Corydalis, and *She Xiang Zhuang Gu Gao* (Plaster for Strengthening Bone Mainly with Moshus) were used in treatment. All of the patients were cured within half a day after treatment started.

Xia Jinling reported 68 cases of stiffneck treated with auricular-point-pressing at Neck (MA－AH10) and Shenmen (MA－TF1). Green gram and *Shang Shi Zhi Tong Gao* (Plaster for Dispelling Dampness and Relieving Pain) or *Huo Xue Zhi Tong Gao* (Plaster for Promoting Blood Circulation to Relieve Pain) were used in treatment. The seeds were pressed for 1 minute with the force increasing gradually to the patient's maximal tolerance. The plasters with stuck seeds were taken off 2 days after the patient's symptoms remitted or disappeared. Result: all of the patients recovered following one treatment session.

2. Acute sprain and contusion

Sprain refers to injury of joints and the soft tissues nearby due to sudden movement of a joint exceeding its normal scope, without fracture, dislocation or skin wound. It is manifested mainly by local pain, swelling and limited movement. The commonly seen are acute sprains of the lumbar region, wrist and ankle.

Contusion refers to injury of soft tissues and subcutaneous hemorrhage in the trunk and limbs resulting from a blunt blow.

TCM holds that sprain and contusion are caused by fall, stumble, contusion, etc. leading to impairment of Channels and Collaterals and stagnation of Qi and Blood.

Point (Fig. 5—36) and method

Main points: Sensitive points in the corresponding area, Subcortex (MA—AT1), Shenmen (MA—TF1), Liver (MA—SC5), Spleen (MA—IC).

Supplementary points: Kidney (MA—SC), Bladder (MA—SC8).

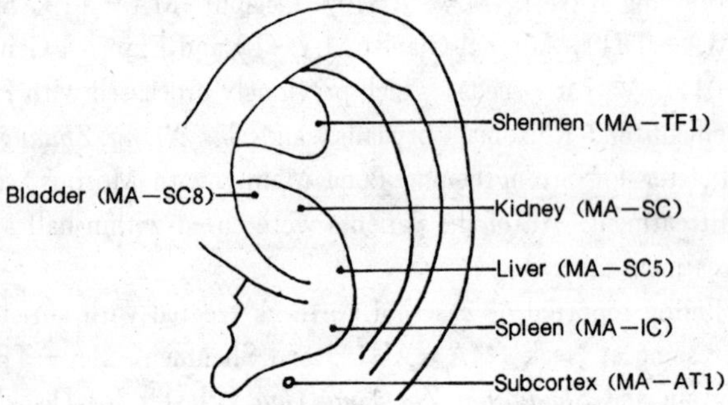

Fig. 5—36 Points for acute sprain and contusion

Method: Apply auricular-point-pressing with vaccaria seeds.

Plaster- sticking therapy with *Huo Xue Zhi Tong Gao* (Plaster for Promoting Blood Circulation to Relieve Pain) or *She Xiang Zhuang Gu Gao* (Plaster for Strengthening Bone Mainly with Moschus) is also applicable. The opposite pressing or perpendicular pressing with strong stimulation is recommended.

Basis for selection of point

Sensitive points in the corresponding area such as Lumbosacral Vertebrae (MA−AH), Wrist (MA−SF2), Ankle (MA−AH2) and Chest (MA−AH10) are selected to promote the flow of Qi and Blood in the local area and dredge Collaterals. Subcortex (MA−AT1) and Shenmen (MA−TF1) are used to tranquilize the mind and relieve pain. Since the Liver dominates the tendons and the Spleen controls the muscles of limbs, Liver (MA−SC5) and Spleen (MA−IC) are selected to relax tendons and muscles, to activate Blood and remove Blood stasis, and to stop pain. In case of acute lumbar sprain, Kidney (MA−SC) and Bladder (MA−SC8) are added.

References for treatment

Liu Shizhong et al reported 1,000 cases of acute joint sprain treated with auricular needling. Among them, 305 were acute lumbar sprain, 45 elbow sprain, 64 wrist sprain, 91 knuckle sprain, 35 knee sprain, and 460 ankle sprain. Points corresponding to the diseased joints and tenderness or sensitive spots are selected as the main points. Needling with filiform needles or embedding with intradermal needles was applied. Following needling, ask the patient to move the affected part. Result: cured in 905 cases (90.5%), improved in 85 cases (8.5%), and ineffective in 10 cases (1%). The total effective rate was 99%.

Yi Guangyu et al reported 100 cases of soft tissue injury treated with finger pressing at auricular points. Corresponding reaction points were selected and treated with finger pressing. Pain was relieved in 66 cases within 10 minutes after treatment started. The total effective rate was 86%.

Shen Zhinu reported 36 cases of acute lumbar sprain treated with plaster-sticking at the following points: Lumbar Vertebrae (MA−

AH), Kidney (MA－SC), Bladder (MA－SC8), Liver (MA－SC5), Shenmen (MA－TF1) and Subcortex (MA－AT1). Vaccaria seeds and *Guan Jie Zhi Tong Gao* (Plaster for relieving Arthralgia) were used for treatment. Press the points until a hot sensation was produced and the pain was reduced. Repeat this procedure again after 1－2 hours. The seeds were taken off 3 days later. Result: cured in 25 cases, improved in 6 cases, and ineffective in 2 cases. The total effective rate was 94.2%.

3. Periarthritis of shoulder

Periarthritis of shoulder is a clinical syndrome marked by soreness, heaviness, pain, limited movement and rigidity of the shoulder. In general, it is considered a chronic inflammatory reaction of the articular cavity and tissues nearby due to retrograde pathological change. This disease occurs mostly in those aged over 40 years, more frequently in female than in male.

The disease is characterized by a slow onset of shoulder pain unilaterally or bilaterally which may radiate to the neck or upper arm and get worse at night, and by an obviously limited movement of the shoulder joint which is severer when the shoulder is in abduction and extorsion. In severe cases with a long duration, there will be muscular atrophy, tissue adhesion and severe dysfunction in the shoulder and arm, while the pain may remit.

TCM terms this disease as *Lou Jian Feng* (Omalgia), *Jian Ning Zheng* (Fronzen Shoulder), *Wu Shi Jian* (Fifty Shoulder), etc.

Point (Fig. 5－37) and method

Main points: Shoulder (MA－SF4), Shoulder Joint (MA), Clavicle (MA－SF5), Shenmen (MA－TF1), Adrenal Gland (MA－AT), Endocrine (MA－IC3).

Supplementary points: Liver (MA－SC5), Spleen (MA－IC).

Method: Apply auricular-point-pressing with vaccaria seeds or plaster- sticking with *Shang Shi Zhi Tong Gao* (Plaster for Dispelling Dampness and Relieving Pain) or *She Xiang Zhuang Gu Gao* (Plaster for Strengthening Bones Mainly with Moschus), or combined use of them. The opposite or perpendicular pressing approach is recommended.

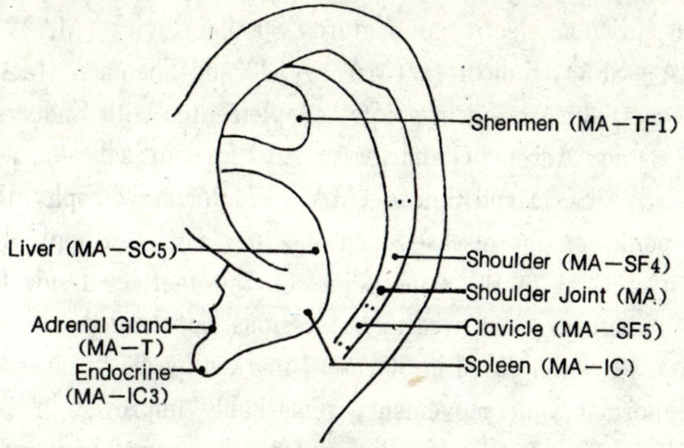

Fig. 5−37 Points for periarthritis of shoulder

As the corresponding points to the diseased part, Shoulder (MA−SF4), Shoulder joint (MA) and Clavicle (MA−SF5) are selected to promote the flow of Qi and Blood, to dredge Channels and to Collaterals, and stop pain. Shenmen (MA−TF1) is for tranquilizing the mind and relieving pain. Since Adrenal Gland (MA−AT) and Endocrine (MA−IC3) have antirheumatic and anti-inflammatory functions, they are used to dispel Wind and dredge Collaterals, relieve inflammation and stop pain to easy joint movement. The Liver stores Blood and dominates tendons while the Spleen governs Blood circulation and controls muscles of the four limbs, so Liver (MA−SC5) and Spleen (MA−IC) are selected and treated with strong stimulation to promote the efficacy of activating Blood and removing its stasis, relaxing tendons and relieving pain.

References for treatment

A report presents 56 cases of periarthritis of shoulder treated with auricular reflex therapy at Shoulder Joint (MA), Clavicle (MA−SF5) and Shenmen (MA−TF1). Direct current was used to stimulate those points in combination with topical application of pepper ointment and massage. After 3−6 months treatment, pain disappeared and motor function of the shoulder joint recovered completely. A follow-up 6 months later showed that 54 cases were cured and 2 improved. The total effective rate was 100%.

Chen Shouji reported 50 cases of periarthritis of shoulder treated with auricular electroacupuncture. Shoulder Joint (MA), Clavicle (MA－SF5), Subcortex (MA－AT1) and Shenmen (MA－TF1) are selected as the main points, supplemented with Endocrine (MA－IC3) and Adrenal Gland (MA－AT) for joint adhesion while Liver (MA－SC5) and Spleen (MA－IC) for amyotrophy. Puncture the points on the diseased side once per day, and apply auricular-point-pressing at the same points on the unaffected side following the puncture. Ten treatment sessions constituted 1 therapeutic course. Result: cured in 30 cases, marked by disappearance of pain and normal joint movement; remarkably improved in 14 cases, marked by obvious pain relief and nearly normal joint movement; mildly improved in 4 cases, marked by reduced pain and ameliorated joint movement; and ineffective in 2 cases. The total effective rate was 96%.

4. Cervical spondylopathy

Cervical spondylopathy, also called cervical spondylotic syndrome, is caused by degeneration of the cervical intervertebral disc and hypersteogeny of the cervical vertebrae. It is characterized by pain of the neck and shoulder, numbness of arms, weakness of muscles, dizziness, cataphlex, abnormal perspiration, staggering gait, even quadriplegia. According to different part oppressed by the diseased cervical vertebrae and subsequent different symptoms, cervical spondylopathy is divided as cervical type, nerve root type, vertebroarterial type, sympathetic type, spinal type and mixed type. The cervical type is mainly manifested as pain in the posterior neck radiating towards the occiput, sensory disturbance or numbness in the occiput. The nerve root type is mainly manifested as pain in the neck and shoulder radiating towards the forearm, and numbness and weakness of the arm. The vertebroarterial type is mainly manifested as dizziness and headache. Cataplexy may occur when the head extends backwards or turns aside suddenly while tinnitus, deafness and nausea may also present. The sympathetic type is mainly manifested as numbness of the limb or part of the face, swelling and coldness of the limbs, abnormal perspiration, arrhythmia and blurred vision. The spinal type is mainly manifested as awkward movement of the limb and unsteady walking with clumsy gait. The mixed type is mainly manifested as symptoms and signs described in two or more types above.

TCM considers that this disease results from deficiency of the Liver and Kidney and from accumulation of Cold leading to stagnation of Qi and Blood and poor nourishment of tendons and muscles.

Point (Fig. 5—38) and method

Main points: Cervical Vertebrae (MA－AH8), Neck (MA－AH10), Kidney (MA—SC), Liver (MA—SC5).

Supplementary points: Shenmen (MA－TF1), Adrenal Gland (MA—AT), Occiput (MA—AT), Heart (MA—IC), Sympathetic (MA—AH7), Spleen (MA—IC).

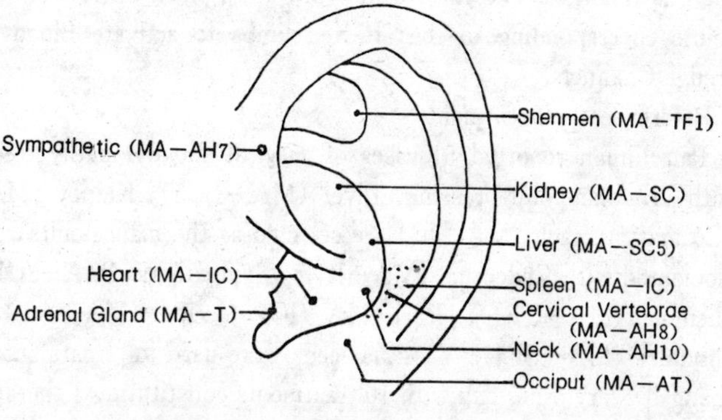

Fig. 5—38 Points for cervical spondylopathy

Method: Apply auricular-point-pressing with vaccaria seeds. For sticking the seeds, *Guan Jie Zhi Tong Gao* (Plaster for Relieving Arthralgia) or *Huo Xue Zhi Tong Gao* (Plaster for Promoting Blood Circulation to Relieve Pain) are applicable. The opposite pressing, perpendicular pressing or intermittent pressing is recommended.

Basis for selection of point

This disease should be treated with the therapeutic principle of replenishing the Liver and Kidney, dredging Channels and Collaterals. As the corresponding points to the diseased part, Cervical Vertebrae

(MA—AH8) and Neck (MA—AH10) are selected to dredge local Channels and Collaterals and promote Blood circulation for the treatment of the Incidental Aspect (Biao) of the disease. Kidney (MA—SC) and Liver (MA—SC5) are used to reinforce the Liver and Kidney, to relax muscles and tendons and strengthen bones for the treatment of the fundamental aspect (Ben) of the disease. For the cervical type, add Occiput (MA—AT) to promote the flow of Qi and Blood in the occipital region. For the nerve root type, add Shenmen (MA—TF1) and Adrenal Gland (MA—AT) to relieve inflammation, spasm and pain and Shoulder (MA—SF4) to activate Channels and Collaterals. For the vertebroarterial type, add Heart (MA—IC) and Occiput (MA—AT) to invigorate Qi and enrich Blood, to tranquilize the mind and relieve dizziness. For the sympathetic type, add Sympathetic (MA—AH7) to regulate vegetative nervous function. For the spinal type, add Spleen (MA—IC) and points corresponding to the affected limbs to activate Blood and dredge Channels.

References for treatment

Pan Jihuan reported 51 cases of cervical spondylopathy treated with auricular-point-pressing. Liver (MA—SC5), Kidney (MA—SC) and Stomach (MA—IC) are selected as the main points, supplemented with Endocrine (MA—IC4), Sympathetic (MA—AH7), Shenmen (MA—TF1), Heart (MA—IC), Occiput (MA—AT) and Shoulder (MA—SF4). Vaccaria seeds were used for treatment and changed every other day with 10 treatments constituting 1 therapeutic course. Result: cured in 30 cases, marked by disappearance of clinical symptoms and no relapse during a one-year follow-up; remarkably improved in 18 cases, marked by approximate disappearance of clinical symptoms and reappearance of mild symptoms following overwork; mildly improved in 3 cases, marked by reduced symptoms and relapse following work. The total effective rate was 100%. Generally, significant efficacy or recovery presented after 10 treatments. Among the 51 cases, the best effect was obtained in the 42 cases of the nerve root type.

Li Daqing et al reported 39 cases of cervical spondylopathy treated with auricular-point-pressing therapy. Among the 39 cases, there were 27 cases of nerve root type, 10 cases of vertebroarterial type, 1 case of cervical type, and 1 case of spinal type. Cervical Vertebrae (MA－AH8), Liver (MA－SC5), Kidney (MA－SC), Spleen (MA－IC), Shenmen (MA－TF1) and Subcortex (MA－AT1) were selected as main points, Occiput (MA—AT) and Internal Ear (MA—L) were supplemented according to the accompanying symptoms. Auricular-point-pressing with vaccaria seeds was applied with opposite or perpendicular pressing approach. For the elderly, auricular massage was adopted. One therapeutic course consisted of 10 treatments. Result: short-term control in 10 cases, marked by short-term disappearance of symptoms; remarkable effect in 27 cases, marked by obvious improvement of symptoms; mild effect in 9 cases, marked by ameliorated symptoms; and no response in 2 cases. The total effective rate was 94.8%.

5. Sciatica

Sciatica is a clinical syndrome, referring to a radiating pain in the distributive area of the sciatic nerve, namely, from the lumbosacral region to the buttocks, the posterior aspect of the thigh, and the posterior-lateral aspect of the shank. The pain is lancinating or burning in nature and usually aggravated by physical activities, sneeze or cough. Physical examinations often find tender spots along the course of sciatic nerve. Lasegue's sign is positive.

According to different causes, sciatica is divided as the primary and the secondary types. The former results from lesion of the sciatic nerve itself due to invasion of Cold-Dampness, inflammation or cold exposure. The latter results from lesion of the adjacent tissues such as prolapse of lumbar vertebral discs, tumor or sacro-iliilis.

The disease mostly occurs in young adults. Its onset is acute or subacute. Primary sciatica has a short course and favorable prognosis.

In TCM, sciatica belongs to the category of *Bi zhen* (Arthralgia). It is considered to be caused by invasion of Wind, Cold and Dampness into Channels and Collaterals leading to stagnation of Channel

Qi.

Point (Fig. 5—39) and method

Mian points: Sciatic Nerve (MA—AH6), Buttocks (MA—AH5), Shenmen (MA—TF1), Subcortex (MA—AT1), Endocrine (MA—IC3), Sympathetic (MA—AH7).

Supplementary points: gallbladder (MA—SC6), Bladder (MA—SC8), Lumbosacral Vertebrae (MA—AH), Kidney (MA—SC).

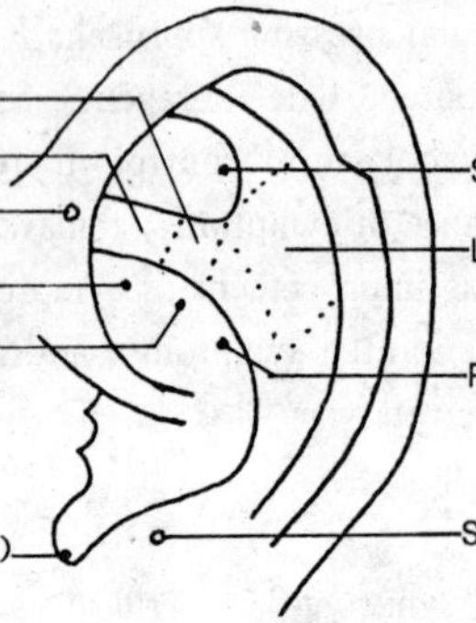

Fig. 5—39 Points for sciatica

Method: Apply auricular-point-pressing with vaccaria seeds. Auricular plaster-sticking method with *She Xiang Zhuang Gu Gao* (Plaster for Strengthening Bones Maily with Moschus), *Xiang Gui Huo Xue Gao* (Plaster for Promoting Blood Circulation Mainly with Moschus and Cortex Cinnamomi) or *Shang Shi Zhi Tong Gao* (Plaster for Dispelling Dampness and Relieving Pain) is also applicable. Therapeutic effects can be improved by combined use of the above two methods. The opposite pressing or perpendicular pressing is recommended.

Basis for selection of point

As the corresponding points to the diseased part, Sciatic Nerve (MA—AH6) and Buttocks (MA—AH5) are selected to dredge Channels and Collaterals. Shenmen (MA—TF1) and Subcortex (MA—AT1) are two important points for tranquilizing the mind and relieving pain. Endocrine (MA—IC3) has antirheumatic and anti-inflammatory functions. Sympathetic (MA—AH7) has the efficacy to expand blood vessels. The joint use of the above points can achieve the therapeutic purpose of dispelling Wind, removing Dampness, activating Blood, dredging Collaterals, and relieving inflammation and pain. If pain mainly affects the lateral aspect of the thigh and shank, which is termed the Shaoyang type, Gallbladder (MA-SC6) should be added. If pain mainly affects the posterior aspect of the thigh and shank, which is termed the Taiyang type, Bladder (MA-SC8) should be added. If there is lumbar vertebral disorder, Lumbosacral Vertebrae (MA-AH) and Kidney (MA-SC) should be added.

References for treatment

Huang Hanxiang reported sciatica treated with auricular needling at Buttocks (MA-AH5), Sciatic Nerve (MA-AH6), Shenmen (MA-TF1), Knee (MA-AH3), Ankle (MA-AH2). Select three of the above points for each treatment, and puncturing them with filiform needles once per day with 10 treatments constituting one therapeutic course. A total effective rate of 98% was obtained.

6. Thromboangiitis obliteans

Thromboangiitis obliteans refers to the segmental inflammatory change of arteries and veins with slow progress. The inflammation of whole strata of Blood vessel leads to hyperplasia of endangium and formation of thrombus with subsequent obliteration of vascular lumen. The severe acro-ischemia then results in acromelic gangrene.

This disease manifests itself by ischemia, numbness and Coldness of extremities, stationary pain and intermittent claudication. In severe case, there may present black and violet color, ulceration, necrosis, even loss of the diseased digits.

In TCM, thromboangiitis obliteans belongs to the category of Tuo Zu (Gangrene of Digits). It is considered to be caused by invasion of Cold and Dampness, emotional disturbance or deficiency of Liver and Kidney, which brings about accumulation of Cold-Dampness, obstruction of Channels and Collaterals, and sluggish flow of Qi and Blood. The onset is also associated with long- term smoking and trauma.

Point (Fig. 5−40) and method

Main points: Heart (MA−IC), Lung (MA−IC1), Liver (MA−SC5), Spleen (MA−IC), Sympathetic (MA−AH7), Endocrine (MA−IC3), Shenmen (MA−TF1).

Supplementary points: Points corresponding to the diseased part, such as Toe (MA−AH) and Finger (MA−SF1), sensitive spots.

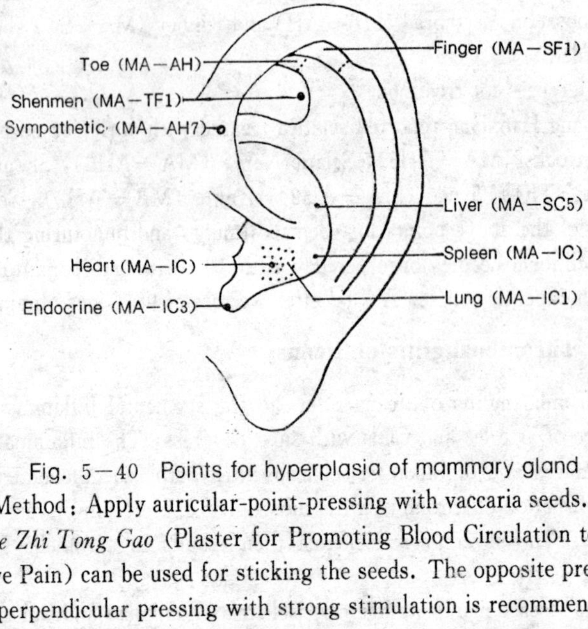

Fig. 5−40 Points for hyperplasia of mammary gland

Method: Apply auricular-point-pressing with vaccaria seeds. *Huo Xue Zhi Tong Gao* (Plaster for Promoting Blood Circulation to Relieve Pain) can be used for sticking the seeds. The opposite pressing or perpendicular pressing with strong stimulation is recommended.

Basis for selection of point

This disease should be treated with the therapeutic principle of invigorating Qi, activating Blood and dredging Collaterals. TCM holds that the Heart governs Blood while the Lung governs Qi. Qi in motion promotes Blood circulation. Therefore, Heart (MA−IC) and Lung (MA−IC1) are selected to invigorate Qi and activate Blood to promote Blood supply of the limb. Since the Liver stores Blood and controls tendons while the Spleen governs Blood to flow within the vessels and dominates limbs and muscles, Liver (MA−

SC5) and Spleen (MA—IC) are used to enrich Blood, to relax muscles and tendons, and to activate Blood for improving nourishment of the limb. Sympathetic (MA—AH7) can regulate vasomotoricity to dilate blood vessels and increase blood supply of the diseased limb. Endocrine (MA—IC3) and Shenmen (MA—TF1) are used to relieve inflammation and pain. The corresponding points to the diseased part, such as Toe (MA—AH) and Finger (MA—SF1), are selected to dredge local Channels. The combined use of the above points can achieve the aim of invigorating Qi, promoting Blood circulation, removing obstruction in Collaterals and relieving pain.

References for treatment

The General Hospital of Chinese People's Liberation Army reported 77 cases of obliterans treated with auricular needling. Points corresponding to the diseased limbs and Warm Point (MA) were selected as main points, supplemented with Sympathetic (MA—AH7), Kidney (MA—SC), Subcortex (MA—AT1), Heart (MA—IC), Lung (MA—IC1), Liver (MA—SC5) and Spleen (MA—IC). One to two of the above points were selected and punctured with filiform needle once per day. Result: basically cured in 6 cases, remarkably improved in 28 cases, pain relieved in 36 cases and failed to respond in 7 cases.

Remarks

Auricular points prove effective for this disease, particularly for relieving pain. However, long-term treatment is needed for improving local symptoms. In clinical practice, Chinese herbal medicine and body acupuncture are often used in combination with auricular acupuncture.

The patient should be advised to give up smoking and keep the affected limb warm.

7. Hyperplasia of mammary gland

Hyperplasia of mammary gland, also called lobular hyperplasia or cystic hyperplasia of the breast, is kind of chronic non-inflammatory and nontumorous mass of the breast, occurring commonly in women between 30—50 years of age. Its onset is associated with dysfunction of the ovary. The patients experience unilateral or bilateral movable masses of varying sizes and irregular forms, which appear simultaneously or successively, and periodic distending pain of the breast, which is closely related to emotion and menstruation.

In TCM, hyperplasia of mammary gland belongs to the category of *Ru Pi* (Nodules of Breast). It is considered to be caused by stagnation of Liver Qi and incoordination between the Liver the and the Stomach leading to accumulation of Phlegm and derangement of Chong and Ren Channels, thus resulting in accumulation of Qi, Blood and Phlegm in the breast and Stomach Channel.

Point (Fig. 5—41) and method

Main points: Chest (MA—AH11), Thoracic Vertebrae (MA—AH8), Liver (MA—SC5), Stomach (MA—SC), Endocrine (MA—IC3), Subcortex (MA—AT1).

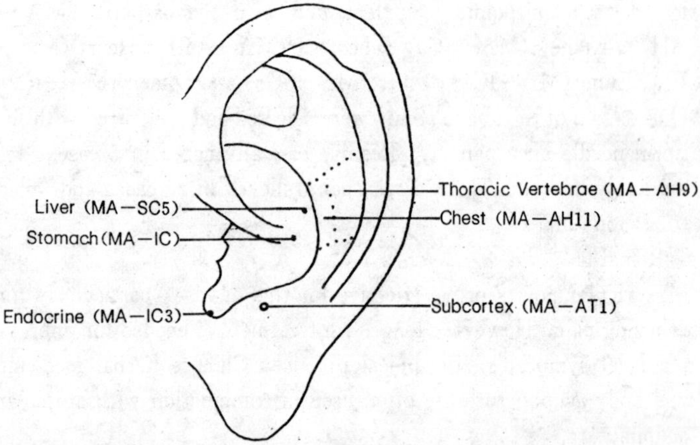

Fig. 5—41 Points for hyperplasia of mammary gland

Method: Apply auricular-point-pressing with vaccaria seeds. *Huo Xue Zhi Tong Gao* (Plaster for Promoting Blood Circulation to Relieve Pain) can be used for sticking the seeds. The opposite pressing or perpendicular pressing with strong stimulation is recommended.

Basis for selection of point

As the corresponding points to the diseased part, Chest (MA—AH11) and Thoracic Vertebrae (MA—AH8) are selected to promote the flow of Qi and Blood in the local Channels and to remove Blood stasis. The Liver governs normal flow of Qi according to TCM knowledge, so Liver (MA－SC5) is used to relieve the depressed Liver. Since the Stomach Channel passes through the breast and abounds in Qi and Blood, Stomach (MA－SC) is adopted to invigorate Qi and activate Blood, to remove Blood stasis and dredge Collaterals. Endocrine (MA－IC3) is used in combination with Subcortex (MA－AT1) to regulate the endocrine function. The joint use of the above points can achieve the purpose of dispersing the stagnant Liver Qi, resolving Phlegm and activating Blood to eliminate masses.

References for treatment

Shen Zhizhong reported 35 cases of nodular hyperplasia of breast treated with auricular-point-pressing mainly at Sympathetic (MA－AH7), Endocrine (MA－IC3), Subcortex (MA－AT1) and Liver (MA－SC5). Vaccaria seeds were used for treatment. Result: after 1－3 treatment courses, cured in 18 cases, marked by disappearance of distending pain and masses; improved in 9 cases, marked by relieved symptoms and reduced masses; and failed to respond in 9 cases. The total effective rate was 76.1%.

Zhang Hehuan reported 15 cases of hyperplasia of mammary gland treated with auricular-point-pressing at Liver (MA－SC5), Stomach (MA－IC) and Chest (MA－AH11). Vaccaria seed or *Xiao Yao Wan* (Easy Pill) was used for treatment and changed once every 3－5 days with 5 times constituting one course. Result: clinically cured in 4 cases, marked by disappearance of distending pain and masses; obviously improved in 5 cases, marked by evident relief of symptoms and masses being reduced by more than a half; mildly improved in 5 cases, marked by relieved symptoms and reduced masses; and failed to respond in 1 case.

8. Urticaria

Urticaria is a localized edema due to dilation and increased osmosis of small vessels caused by various factors. It is clinically divided as the cutaneous type and the gastrointestinal type. Cutaneous urticaria is mainly manifested as a sudden onset of wheals varying in size and form, accompanied with intolerable itching. The wheals, pink or pale in color, develop in number and size from point-like to patch-like, while they disappear without any trace. The gastrointestinal urticaria is manifested as abdominal pain, diarrhea, vomiting, nausea and dyspnea.

The urticaria with recovery within several days to several weeks is defined as the acute type, while that with repeated attacks lasting over one month, sometimes severe, sometimes mild, is defined as the chronic type.

TCM terms this disorder as *Feng Tuan Kuai* (Wheal), *Yin Zhen* (Hidden Rash), or *Chi Bai You Feng* (Pink or White Migratory Wind-Syndrome). It is considered to be caused by improper diet such as over intake of meat, fish or alcohol which impairs the Spleen and Stomach in transporting and transforming nutrients, leading to retention of Dampness-Heat. It can also be caused by invasion of Cold, Wind, Dampness and Heat into the skin portion due to weak constitution. The failure of the defensive Qi to protect the body from diseases and the insufficiency of Blood to nourish the skin will bring about the occurrence of urticaria.

Point (Fig. 5—42) and method

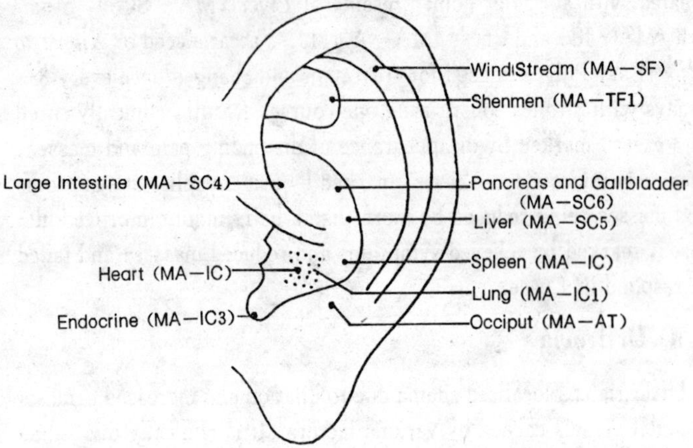

Fig. 5—42 Points for urticaria

Main points: Lung (MA－IC1), Wind Stream (MA－SF), Adrenal Gland (MA－AT), Endocrine (MA－IC3), Shenmen (MA－TF1).

Supplementary points: Ear Apex (MA－H6), Stomach (MA－IC), Large Intestine (MA－SC4), Small Intestine (MA－SC2).

Method: Apply auricular-point-pressing with vaccaria seeds or magnetic beads. The opposite pressing or perpendicular pressing is recommended.

Basis for selection of point

The Lung is in charge of the skin and hair, therefore, Lung (MA－IC1) is selected to disperse the defensive Qi, to dispel Wind and relieve superficial syndrome. Wind Stream (MA－SF) has antirheumatic and anti-inflammatory functions. According to Western medicine, Endocrine (MA－IC3) is selected to promote secretion of various active hormones, and Adrenal Gland (MA－AT) to increase adrenocortical hormones while inhibit the release of histamine to suppress dermal antigen-antibody reaction and exudation of capillary. Shenmen (MA－TF1) is used to tranquilize the mind and relieve itching. The joint use of the above points can achieve the purpose of dispelling Wind, activating Blood, tranquilizing the mind and checking itching. In case of the gastrointestinal type, Stomach (MA－IC), Large Intestine (MA－SC4) and Small Intestine (MA－SC2) are added. In case of acute stage, Ear Apex (MA－H6) is added and treated with bloodletting method.

References for treatment

Yi Zhenyun reported 25 cases of intractable urticaria treated with auricular-point-pressing, of which the shortest disease duration was 7 days while the longest 2 years. Points selected were: Lung (MA－IC1), Adrenal Gland (MA－AT), Endocrine (MA－IC3), Shenmen (MA－TF1) and Wind Stream (MA－SF). Green gram and zinc oxide tape were used for treatment once every 4 days. Result: 5, 8, 6, 3 and 3 cases were cured respectively after 2, 3, 4, 6 and 7 treatments.

Zhao Yongming et al reported 121 cases of urticaria treated with auricular-point-pressing. Points used were Shenmen (MA－TF1),

Heart (MA−IC), Lung (MA−IC1), Wind Stream (MA−SF), Subcortex (MA−AT1), Spleen (MA−IC), Stomach (MA−IC) and Ear Apex (MA−H6). Vaccaria seeds were used for treatment and changed twice per week with 5−10 treatment sessions constituting one therapeutic course. After a mean treatment of 7 sessions, 35 cases were cured, 41 cases were remarkably improved, 34 cases were mildly improved, and 11 cases failed to respond. The total effective rate was 90.91%.

9. Cutaneous pruritis

Cutaneous pruritis is a kind of the dermotosis, manifested as itching and subsequent skin injury without primary lesion, occurring commonly in elderly and middle-aged people. It is divided as a general type and a localized type. The general type is characterized by a paroxysmal and wandering itching throughout the body. The itching may be different in severity in different individuals. However, it usually gets worse at night and badly disturbs the patient's sleep since it has to be relieved by continuous scratching until the skin bleeds and pain arises instead. This disease is often induced or aggravated by emotional disturbances, drinking of alcohol, taking of irritant food, exposure to hot or cold, or rub of the skin by clothes. The localized itching is characterized by limited itching in one part of the body such as the anus, vulva, head and leg.

In TCM, cutaneous pruritis belongs to the categories of *Yang Feng* (Itch Wind-Syndrome) and *Feng Sao Yang* (Itching due to Wind). It is considered to be caused by invasion of Cold, Dampness or Heat into the Lung and the Muscular Striae due to deficiency of the Lung Qi failing to defend the body, or caused by deficiency of the Kidney Yin and the Liver Yin and insufficiency of Blood resulting in malnutrition of the skin.

Point (Fig. 5−43) and method

Main points: Points corresponding to the diseased part, Lung (MA−IC1) Large Intestine (MA−SC4), Wind Stream (MA−SF), Endocrine (MA−IC3), Shenmen (MA−TF1), Occiput (MA−AT).

Supplementary points: Liver (MA—SC5), Spleen (MA—IC), Heart (MA—IC), Pancreas and Gallbladder (MA—SC6).

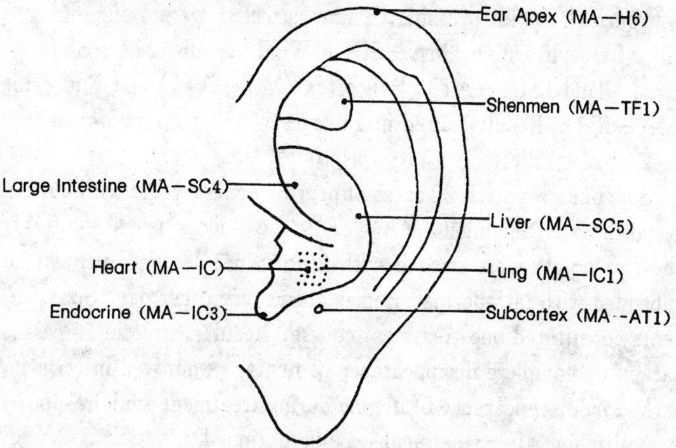

Fig. 5—43 Points for cutaneous pruritis

Method: Apply auricular-point-pressing with vaccaria seeds. It can also be combined with pricking the corresponding points to cause bleeding. The perpendicular pressing with strong stimulation is recommended.

Basis for selection of point

Points corresponding to the diseased part are selected to promote the flow of Qi and Blood, to dispel Wind and dredge Collaterals. The Lung governs the skin and hair and is associated with the Large Intestine, therefore, Lung (MA—IC1) and Large Intestine (MA—SC4) are selected to disperse the Lung Qi, to dispel Wind and relieve itching. Wind Stream (MA—SF) and Endocrine (MA—IC3) are used to dispel Wind, to stop itching and resist allergic reaction. Shenmen (MA—TF1) and Occiput (MA—AT) are employed to tranquilize the mind and arrest itching. In case of itching in elderly people with Blood deficiency, Heart (MA—IC), Liver (MA—SC5) and Spleen (MA—IC) are added. In case of itching resulting from jaundice, Liver (MA—SC5) and Pancreas and Gallbladder (MA—SC6) are added. In case of diabetic pruritis, Pancreas and Gallbladder (MA—SC6) is added.

References for treatment

Zheng Guangliang reported 30 cases of cutaneous pruritis treated with auricular-point-pressing. Points selected were Lung (MA—IC1), Large Intestine (MA—SC4), Wind Stream (MA—SF), Adrenal Gland (MA—AT), Subcortex (MA—AT1) and Endocrine (MA—IC3). Result: cured in 28 cases (93.33%), improved in 2 cases. The total effective rate was 100%.

Luo Yumin reported 30 cases of pruritis snilis treated with auricular needling at Shenmen (MA—TF1) and Endocrine (MA—IC3). The two points were treated with filiform needles once per day or embedded with intradermal needles once every other day. Six treatments constituted one treatment course. Result: cured in 25 cases, marked by complete disappearance of itching; improved in 5 cases, marked by disappearance of itching during treatment while reappearance of itching after treatment was discontinued.

10. Neurodermatitis

Neurodermatitis is a kind of chronic inflammatory dermatosis characterized by paroxysmal severe itching, lichenoid change of the skin and a close relation with psyche and emotion. In Western medicine, its etiology remains unclear. It is considered to be associated with the imbalance of excito-inhibitory function of the cerebral cortex. Mental stress, over fatigue and mechanical stimulation may induce onset of the disease. Skin lesion frequently appears in the neck, limbs such as the elbow, popliteal fossa, interior side of the thigh and extensor aspect of the forearm. In case of neurodermatitis developing in the four limbs, the skin lesion, mostly symmetrically distributed, is a kind of irregular polygonal flat papulae of the miliary size, which are distributed in line with the wrinkles of the skin and may merge into lichenoid change with dry surface and itching sensation.

In TCM, neurodermatitis is similar to *Niu Pi Xuan* (Cowskin Tinea or Psoriasis) because the affected skin looks like the cowhide, thick and hard. It is considered to be caused by invasion of Wind,

Dampness and Heat into the skin, which will produce Heat and dryness after prolonged stagnation and subsequently lead to poor nourishment of the skin.

Point (Fig. 5—44) and method

Main points: Points corresponding to the diseased part, Lung (MA—IC1), Subcortex (MA—AT1), Endocrine (MA—IC3), Shenmen (MA—TF1).

Supplementary points: Ear Apex (MA—H6), Heart (MA—IC), Large Intestine (MA—SC4), Liver (MA—SC5).

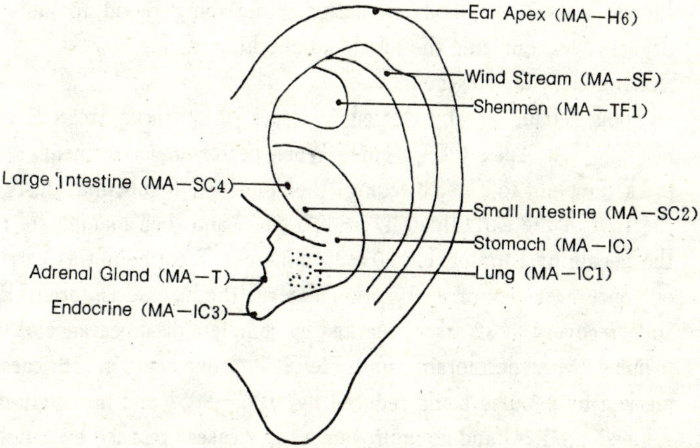

Fig. 5—44 Points for neurodermatitis

Method: Mostly apply auricular-point-pressing with vaccaria seeds. The perpendicular pressing approach is recommended. Ear Apex (MA—H6) is usually pricked to cause bleeding.

Basis for selection of point

Points corresponding to the diseased part are selected to promote the flow of Qi and Blood in the local area and dredge Channels. Lung (MA—IC1) is used to facilitate the flow of the Lung Qi, to dispel Wind and clear away Heat. Subcortex (MA—AT1) is used to regulate the excito-inhibitory function of the cerebral cortex and the function of the vegetative nerve. Endocrine (MA—IC3) and Shenmen (MA—TF1) are employed to relieve inflammation, to dispel

Wind, to enrich and activate Blood, to tranquilize the mind and arrest itching. Ear Apex (MA—H6) treated with pricking treatment is added to strengthen the efficacy of dispelling Wind and clearing away Heat from the Blood. The Lung and the Large Intestine are interiorly-exteriorly related, Large Intestine (MA—SC4) is therefore added to improve the function of the Lung (MA—IC1) in dispersing the Lung Qi, dispelling Wind and clearing away Heat. Heart (MA—IC) and Liver (MA—SC5) are added to enrich and activate Blood as well as to purge Fire and relieve depression. The joint use of the above points can reach the purpose of clearing away Heat to cool Blood, activating Blood circulation, nourishing Blood to moisten dryness, tranquilizing the mind and checking itching.

References for treatment

Zhou Zeliang et al reported 50 cases of psoriasis treated with needling Ear Apex (MA—H6). When performing treatment, first prick the point to cause bleeding, then puncture it subcutaneously to the root of the ear (about 1.5—2.5 cm), and then manipulate the the needle by rotating for 20—30 minutes. Treatment was carried out once everyday or every other day till the disease is cured. Result: recovery in 32 cases, marked by complete disappearance of the papulae with decolorant spots left; improvement in 16 cases, marked by papulae being reduced by 50%—90% and no newly-developed papulae; and no improvement in 2 cases, marked by papulae being reduced less than 30% and newly-developed papulae after three-week treatment.

11. Flat wart

Flat wart is a kind of viral dermotosis. Because flat wart occurring commonly in young people, it is also called youth wart. Flat wart is clinically manifested as relatively rapid onset of papulae mostly in the face and on the dorsum of the hand and forearm. The papula is pin-point or rice-grain like in size, round or irregular in form, light brown, pink or normal in color, and smooth and hard with definite border in structure. Patients suffering from this disease have no subjective symptoms or only slight itching. The papulae may withdraw automatically without leaving any scar behind but may recur later. The duration of disease may be prolonged from several months to several years.

In TCM, flat wart is considered to be caused by attack of blended Wind and Dampness in the skin, or hyperactivity of the Liver Fire triggered by anger leading to consumption of Blood and stagnation of Qi and Blood.

Point (Fig. 5—45) and method

Main points: Lung (MA—IC1), Large Intestine (MA—SC4), Shenmen (MA—TF1), Subcortex (MA—AT1), Endocrine (MA—IC3).

Supplementary points: Points corresponding to the diseased part, Ear Apex (MA—H6), Liver (MA—SC5), Stomach (MA—IC).

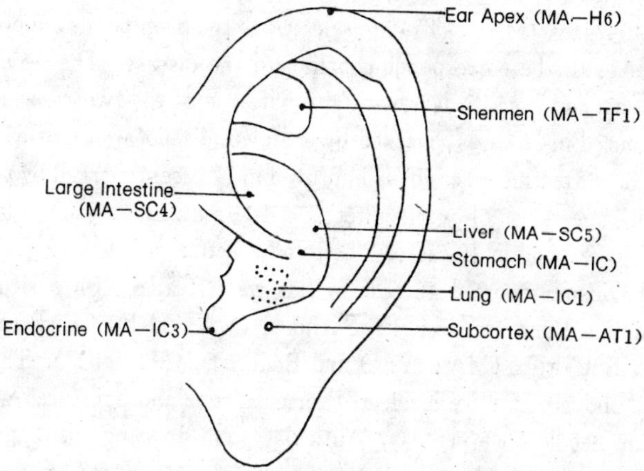

Fig. 5—45 Points for flat wart

Method: Mostly apply auricular-point-pressing with vaccaria seeds. The opposite pressing or perpendicular pressing is recommended.

Basis for selection of point

Since the Lung controls the skin and hair and is exteriorly-interiorly related with the Large Intestine, Lung (MA—IC1) and Large Intestine (MA—SC4) are selected to promote the dispersing function of the Lung Qi and activate the flow of Qi and Blood to ensure the normal state of the skin. Shenmen (MA－TF1), Subcortex (MA－AT1) and Endocrine (MA－IC3) are used to tranquilize and calm the mind, to relieve itching and regulate endocrine function to promote body metabolism. Points corresponding to the diseased part are added to dredge the local Channels and eliminate pathogenic Heat. In case of the blended Wind, Heat and Toxin in the skin, Ear Apex (MA－H6) is added and treated with pricking method to clear away Heat and Toxic Materials. In case of hyperactivity of the Liver with Blood deficiency, Liver (MA－SC5) and Stomach (MA－IC) are added to nourish Yin for moistening Dryness.

References for treatment

Qiu Zaijing reported 102 cases of youth wart treated with intradermal- needle-embedding. Lung (MA－IC1), Stomach (MA－IC) and Subcortex (MA－AT1) are selected as the main points, supplemented with the corresponding points to the disease. The needles were changed every 3 days with alternate use of the two ears. Result: cured in 75 cases, marked by complete disappearance of warts after 3－6 treatment sessions; improved in 17 cases, marked by partial disappearance of warts after 7－10 treatment sessions; and failed to respond in 10 cases. The total effective rate was 90%.

Da Qiusun reported 46 case of flat wart treated with auricular needling at Lung (MA－IC1), Shenmen (MA－TF1), Cheek (MA－L), Subcortex (MA－AT1) and Endocrine (MA－IC3). Three of the above points were selected for each time and punctured with filiform needle once per day. Auricular-point-pressing was applied for those who could not make it to come to hospital for treatment every day. Result: basically cured in 8 cases, remarkably improved in 8 cases, mildly improved in 23 cases, and failed to response in 7 cases. The total effective rate was 84.8%.

12. Herpes zoster

Herpes zoster is a kind of viral dermatosis, frequently seen in spring and autumn. It is clinically manifested as feverish, itching and tight sensation of the diseased area in the beginning, which progresses to red spots and grouped blisters of the size from a millet to a rice-grain or green gram. The blisters contain clear or turbid fluid and distribute along the peripheral nerves, mostly in the distributive area of unilateral intercostal nerve or trigeminal nerve. Other symptoms may include burning sensation, severe pain, or even mild fever, insomnia and swelling of the nearby lymph nodes. If there is no secondary infection, the erosive surface of the broken blister will be dry and form a scab several days later. Pigmentation and shallow scar are left temporarily after recovery.

In TCM, herpes zoster belongs to the categories of *She Dan* (Snake- Shaped Rash) and *Chan Yao Huo Dan* (Heat Rash Belching the Waist). It is considered to be caused mostly by hyperactivity of the Liver Fire and internal accumulation of Dampness-Heat, or caused by invasion of blended Dampness-Heat in the skin.

Point (Fig. 5—46) and method

Main points: Points corresponding to the diseased part, Ear apex (MA—H6), Lung (MA—IC1), Liver (MA—SC5), Pancreas and Gallbladder (MA—SC6), Endocrine (MA—IC3).

Supplementary points: Shenmen (MA—TF1), Subcortex (MA—AT1).

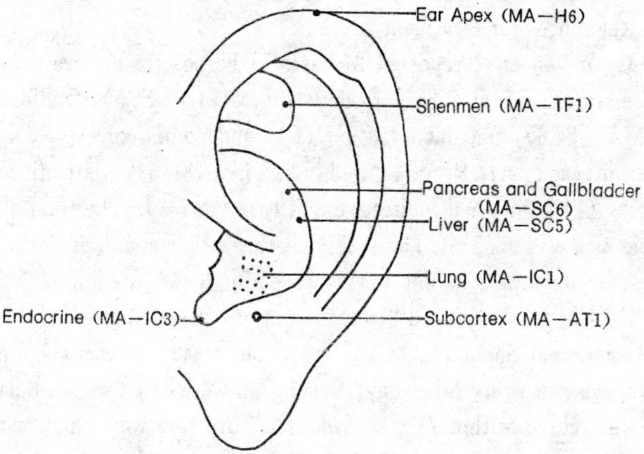

Fig. 5—46 Points for herpes zoster

Method: Mostly apply auricular-point-pressing with vaccaria seeds or Borneo. The opposite pressing or perpendicular pressing is recommended.

Basis for selection of point

This disease should be treated with therapeutic principles of clearing away Heat, Dampness and Toxic Materials, activating Blood, dredging Channels and relieving pain. Points corresponding to the diseased part are selected to activate Blood, to dredge Channels and relieve pain. Ear apex (MA−H6) is treated with pricking method for clearing away Heat, Dampness and Toxic Materials. Lung (MA−IC1) is used to relieve superficial syndrome and eliminate Heat. Liver (MA−SC5) and Pancreas and Gallbladder (MA−SC6) are used to remove Dampness-Heat from the Liver and Gallbladder. Endocrine (MA−IC3) has anti-inflammatory function and therefore is employed to promote discharge of the Toxic Materials, to eliminate Dampness and stop pain. In case of severe pain, Shenmen (MA−TF1) and Subcortex (MA−AT1) are added to tranquilize the mind and relieve pain. The joint use of the points can achieve the purpose of clearing away Heat, Toxic Materials and Dampness. As a result, the red spot disappears, the blister dries, and the pain remits due to smooth flow of Qi and Blood in the Channels.

References for treatment

Guan Fen et al reported 27 cases of herpes zoster treated with laser irradiation at auricular points Liver (MA−SC5), Gallbladder (MA−SC6), Shenmen (MA−TF1) and points corresponding to the diseased part. Result: cured in 22 cases (81.5%), effective in 4 cases (14.8%), and ineffective in 1 case (3.7%). The total effective rate was 96.3%. The author of this article also found that the cellular immune function was improved in all the cured patients.

Cai Chengsui reported 27 cases of herpes zoster treated with laser irradiation at Shenmen (MA−TF1). The treatment was given once every day or every other day. Result: 22 were cured within 6 days, 5 were cured within 7−12 days. The cure rate was 100% with a mean course of treatment of 6.5 days.

13. Chloasma

Chloasma is a skin disease characterized by yellowish brown patches in the face. It is also called "butterfly patch" since the form of the patch resembles a butterfly. Chloasma occurs commonly in young adults, particularly in women. Its main clinical manifestations are yellowish brown or dark brown patches with a smooth surface and a definite but irregular border in the face and absence of subjective symptoms. The patches are usually symmetrically distributed in the cheek like a map or butterfly, sometimes involving the forehead, zygomatic region, nose, perioral region or mental region.

TCM terms this disorder as *Li Hei Ban* (Dark Patch). It is believed to be caused by deficiency of the Kidney with depression of the Liver Qi and incoordination between Qi and Blood, resulting in Blood stasis.

Point (Fig. 5—47) and method

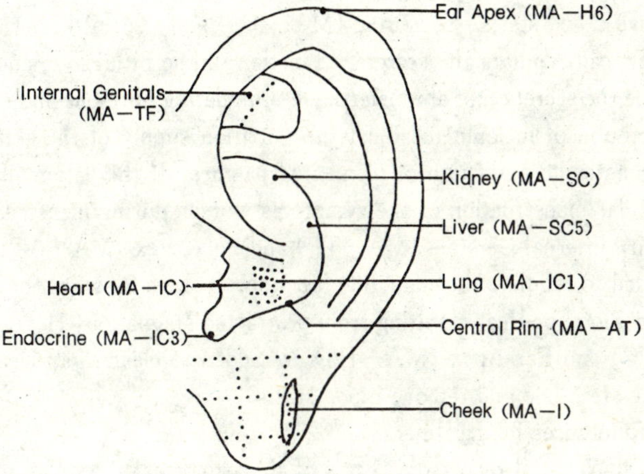

Fig. 5—47 Points for chloasma

Main points: Cheek (MA—L), Lung (MA—IC1), Liver (MA—SC5), Kidney (MA—SC), Endocrine (MA—IC3), Central Rim (MA—AT).

Supplementary points: Internal Genitals (MA-TF), Heart (MA-IC), Ear Apex (MA-H6).

Method: Apply auricular-point-pressing with vaccaria seeds. *Huo Xue Zhi Tong Gao* (Plaster for Promoting Blood Circulation to Relieve Pain) and *Xiang Gui Huo Xue Gao* (Plaster for Promoting Blood Circulation Mainly with Moschus and Cortex Cinnamomi) can be used for sticking the seeds. The opposite pressing or intermittent pressing is recommended.

Basis for selection of point

This disease should be treated with the therapeutic principle of promoting the flow of Qi and Blood and removing Blood stasis to eliminate patches. Since the Lung controls the skin, Lung (MA-IC1) is selected in combination with Cheek (MA-L), a corresponding point to the diseased part, to promote the flow of Qi and Blood, to remove Blood stasis and eliminate patches. The Liver stores Blood while the Kidney stores Essence, Liver (MA-SC5) and Kidney (MA-SC) are therefore used to relieve the depressed Liver and replenish the Kidney Essence, to activate Blood and remove Blood stasis. Endocrine (MA-IC3) and Central Rim (MA-AT) can regulate the secretary function of the pituitary gland, induce the secretion of antimelanocyte-stimulating hormone and reduce secretion of melanin to adjust the nutrition supply of the skin and promote the extinction of pigmented patches. If the patient has irregular menstruation or the symptoms worsen during menstrual period, Internal Genitals (MA-TF) and Subcortex (MA-AT1) are added to regulate the endocrine function. If there is stagnation of Qi and Blood or Heat resulting from protracted stagnation, Heart (MA-IC) and Ear Apex (MA-H6) are added to clear away Heat, to activate Blood and remove Blood stasis.

References for treatment

Du Wei et al reported 50 cases of chloasma treated with auricular-lar-point-pressing. Main points used were Shenmen (MA-TF1), Internal Genitals (MA-TF), Liver (MA-SC5), Kidney (MA-SC), Spleen (MA-IC), Endocrine (MA-IC3) and Subcortex (MA-AT1). Vaccaria seeds were used and the stuck seeds were changed every other day with 15 treatment sessions constituting one course. Medicines were discontinued during this treatment. Result: remarkable effect in 26 cases, marked by obvious improvement of pigmentation and related symptoms; medium effect in 15 cases, marked by clear discoloration of pigmentation and improvement of related symptoms; mild effect in 7 cases, marked by discoloration of pigmentation and improvement of related symptoms; and inefficacy in 2 cases. The total effective rate was 96%.

Shi Yian reported 80 cases of chloasma treated with auricular-point- pressing. Main points used were Liver (MA−SC5), Kidney (MA−SC), Lung (MA−IC1), Endocrine (MA−IC3), Subcortex (MA−AT1), Sympathetic (MA−AH7) and Cheek (MA−L). The vaccaria seeds were used and changed every other day with 10 treatment sessions constituting one course. Result: excellent efficacy in 36 cases (45%), marked by disappearance of pigmentation after one course of treatment; good efficacy in 38 cases (47. 5%), marked by obvious extinction of pigmentation after two courses of treatment; and unsatisfactory efficacy in 6 cases (7. 5%), marked by no evident extinction of pigmentation.

14. Acne

Acne refers to an inflammation occurring in hair follicle and sebaceous glands. It is clinically characterized by comedo, papula, pustula and nodule in the face or on the chest and back, which occurs mostly in adolescents. Acne is simply divided as the shallow type and the deep type. The shallow type only presents papule or pustule, which can suppurate quickly and then be absorbed naturally. This process is short and densely- distributed small black spots are left after it. The deep type presents bead-sized or even bigger dark red and hard nodules with obvious inflammation and infiltration. Generally the nodules do not suppurate. Acne is usually caused by endocrine changes in adolescent leading to hypersteatosis and subsequently obstruction of the excretory pores. Invasion of bacteria contributes to its occurrence.

In TCM, acne belongs to the category of *Fei Feng Fen Ci* (Lung-

Wind Comedo). It is also called *Mian Pi Bao* (Facial Papula) or *Fei Feng Bao* (Lung-Wind Eruption). Acne is considered to be caused by retention of Heat in the Lung and Stomach steaming the face and resulting in the stagnation of Qi and Blood.

Point (Fig. 5—48) and method

Main points: Lung (MA—IC1), Large Intestine MA—SC4), Stomach (MA—IC), Ear Apex (MA—H6), Endocrine (MA—IC3), Subcortex (MA—AT1), corresponding points to the diseased part.

Supplementary point: Shenmen (MA—TF1).

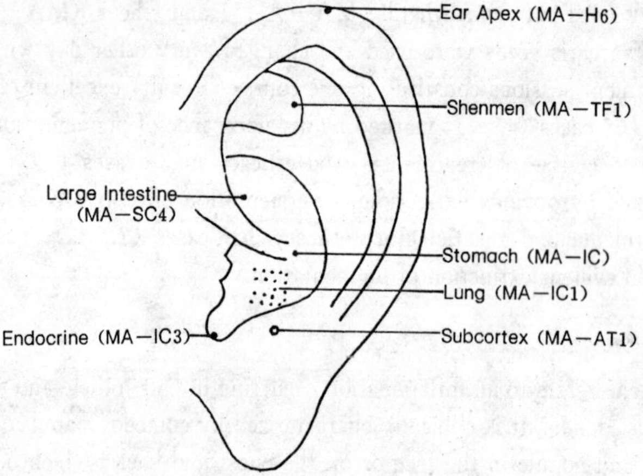

Fig. 5—48 Points for acne

Method: Apply auricular-point-pressing with vaccaria seeds or green grams, or in combination with plaster-sticking therapy. The opposite pressing or perpendicular pressing is recommended.

Basis for selection of point

Points corresponding to the diseased part are used in combination with Lung (MA—IC1), Large Intestine MA—SC4) and Stomach (MA—IC) to clear away Heat from the Lung and the Stomach. Ear Apex (MA—H6) has the function of purging Heat and removing Blood stasis, therefore it is combined with Endocrine (MA—IC3) and Subcortex (MA—AT1) to regulate endocrine and metabolism of sebum and promote the flow of Qi and Blood throughout the body, thus promoting extinction of acne. In case of itching sensation, Ear Apex (MA—H6) is added to tranquilize the mind and arrest itching.

References for treatment

Zhang Huanan reported 50 cases of acne treated with auricular-point- pressing therapy. The main points used were Lung (MA—IC1), Shenmen (MA—TF1), Sympathetic (MA—AH7) and Subcortex (MA—AT1). The vaccaria seeds were used for treatment with 5 treatment sessions constituting one course. Result: 12, 17, 13, 5 cases were cured after 1, 2, 3, 4 treatment courses respectively. The total cure rate was 94%. The remaining 3 cases were improved. A total effective rate of 100% was obtained.

Xu Mingyu reported 381 cases of acne treated with auricular cutting therapy. Lung (MA—IC1) was used as the main point, supplemented with Shenmen (MA—TF1), Sympathetic (MA—AH7), Endocrine (MA—IC3) and Subcortex (MA—AT1). Method: after routine sterilization, slightly cut the skin of the selected points with a surgical knife blade to let out a little Blood and then apply prepared medicinal powder to the treated area to prevent infection. The powder consisted of equal amount of triturated realgar, borneol, peppermint and talcum powder and was mixed with the same amount of boric acid. Treatment was performed once every other day with 10 treatment sessions constituting one course. Result: 94, 136, 96, 29 cases were cured after 1, 2, 3, 4, treatment course, respectively. The total cure rate was 94%.

15. Phantom limb pain

Phantom limb pain is a psychic disease manifested as a feeling of existence and pain at the limb which has lost due to trauma or amputation. The pain may be severe with a nature of electric shock, lancinating, tearing or burning, which is persistent but aggravated at times. It often occurs following secondary injury or psychic stimulation.

Modern medicine believes that phantom is associated with central nervous system. After amputation, the inhibitory impulse of nonspecific pain on the spinal is reduced, subsequently leading to an abnormal increase of the pain excitability.

TCM holds that disorder of the Channel Qi due to broken of the Channels after amputation causes stagnation of Qi and Blood and obstruction of Channels, thus leading to pain.

Point (Fig. 5—49) and method

Main points: Points corresponding to the diseased part, such as Toe (MA—AH) and Finger (MA—SF1), Subcortex (MA—AT1), Adrenal Gland (MA—T), Shenmen (MA—TF1).

Supplementary points: Occiput (MA—AT), Anterior Ear Lobe (MA—L), Ear Apex (MA—H6).

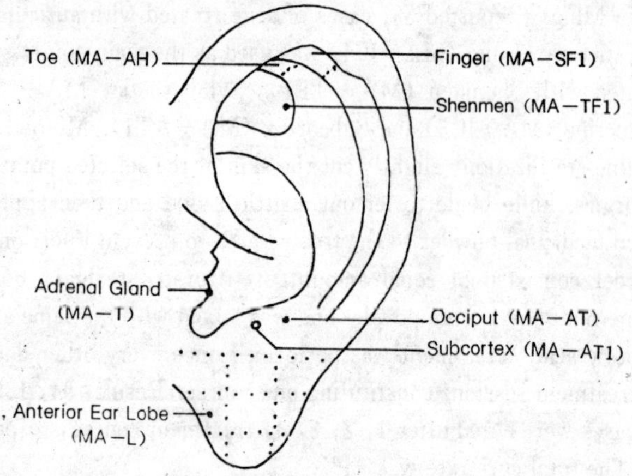

Fig. 5—49 Points for phantom limb pain

Method: Apply auricular-point-pressing with vaccaria seeds or magnetic beads. The opposite pressing or perpendicular pressing is recommended.

Basis for selection of point

Points corresponding to the diseased part are selected to regulate the local Channel Qi, activate Blood and remove Blood stasis. What's more, by stimulating those points to induce a new focus of excitation, the previous hyperexcitation of the cerebral cortex which elicits phantom limb pain is relieved. Subcortex (MA—AT1) is used to regulate the excito-inhibitory function of the cerebral cortex. Adrenal Gland (MA－T) can regulate nerves and blood vessels. Shenmen (MA－TF1) is used to tranquilize the mind and stop pain. The joint use of the above points can achieve the purpose of dredging Channels and Collaterals, promoting the flow of Qi and Blood, removing Blood stasis and relieving pain. For severe pain that disturbs sleep, Occiput (MA－AT) and Anterior Ear Lobe (MA－L) are added. For severe pain accompanied with warm sensation, Ear Apex (MA－H6) is added and treated with pricking method to cause bleeding.

References for treatment

Liu Guiliang reported 13 cases of limb hallucinosis treated with intradermal-needle-embedding at Shenmen (MA－TF1), Subcortex (MA－AT1), Adrenal Gland (MA－T) and points corresponding to the diseased part. The treatment was given once per 3－5 days. After treatment, all of the patients were cured.

16. Erythromelagia

Erythromelagia is a vascular disease characterized by paroxysmal temperature increase, redness, swelling and severe burning pain in the skin of the extremities, especially in the sole and toes. The increase of environment temperature can aggravate this burning pain. Work and sleep may be disturbed in severe cases.

Erythromelagia mostly occurs in young adults. Although the etiology remains unclear, it is considered to be related to dysfunction of the central nerve and vegetative nerve leading to peripheral vasomotor ataxia and hyperdilation of small arteries in the extremities, and subsequently causing disturbance of local Blood flow and local congestion.

In TCM, erythromelagia belongs to the category of *Xue Bi* (Blood Bi Syndrome) and *Yu Xue* (Blood Stasis).

Point (Fig. 5－50) and method

Main points: Sympathetic (MA－AH7), Shenmen (MA－TF1), Subcortex (MA－AT1), Points corresponding to the diseased part, such as Toe (MA－AH) and Finger (MA－SC1).

Supplementary points: Occiput (MA－AT), Anterior Ear Lobe (MA－L).

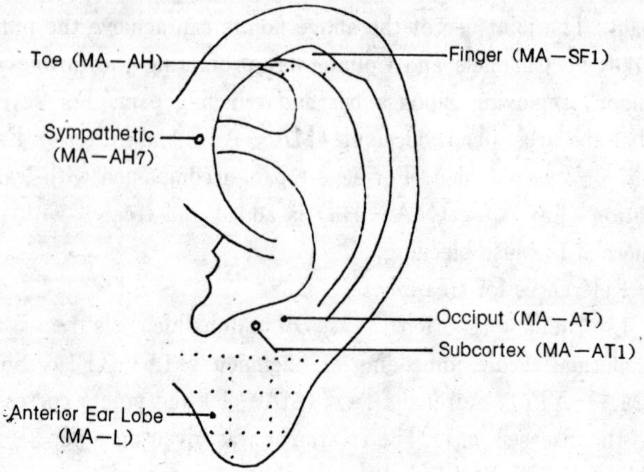

Fig. 5－50 Points for erythromelagia

Method: Mostly apply auricular-point-pressing with vaccaria seeds or magnetic beads. *She Xiang Zhuang Gu Gao* (Plaster for Strengthening Bones Mainly with Moschus) or *Xiang Gui Huo Xue Gao* (Plaster for Promoting Blood Circulation with Moschus and Cortex Cinnamomi) can be used for sticking the seeds. The opposite pressing or perpendicular pressing is recommended.

Basis for selection of point

According to Western medicine, Sympathetic (MA－AH7) and Subcortex (MA－AT1) are selected to regulate the vegetative nerve and vasomotoricity. Shenmen (MA－TF1) is used to tranquilize the mind and relieve pain. Points corresponding to the diseased part are employed to dredge local Channels and regulate Qi and Blood to stop pain. In case of poor sleep due to severe pain, Occiput (MA－AT) and Anterior Ear Lobe (MA－L) are added.

Remarks

Auricular acupuncture proves quite effective for improving symptoms of this disease. However, the patients should be asked to persist in this treatment until symptoms are under control.

During the period of treatment, the patients should avoid taking irritant diet such as sour, pungent food and alcohol, avoid exposure to cold and over fatigue, and avoid use of vasodilator.

17. Postoperative abdominal distension

Because of paralysis of the gastrointestinal smooth muscle due to operation, the patient may feel abdominal distension or even difficulty in breathing due to elevation of the diaphragm. Pulmonary complications may develop in some cases. In addition, severe abdominal distension can affect the healing of the gastroenteric stoma and the wound on the abdominal wall.

Postoperative abdominal distension occurs mostly following operations of the abdominal cavity, pelvis or spine. It is caused by inhibited gastrointestinal peristalsis due to stimulation on the gastrointestine or its nerves, or due to hypokalemia.

Point (Fig. 5—51) and method

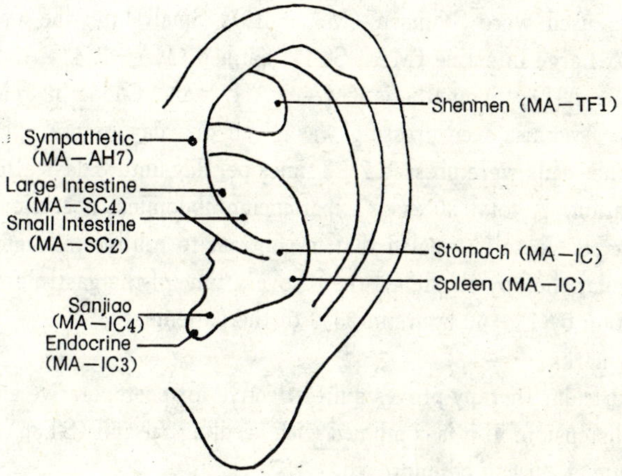

Fig. 5—51 Points for postperative abdominal distension

Main points: Large Intestine (MA—SC4), Small Intestine (MA—SC2), Spleen (MA—IC), Stomach (MA—IC), Sympathetic (MA—AH7), Sanjiao (MA—IC4).

Supplementary points: Shenmen (MA—TF1), Endocrine (MA—IC3).

Method: Mostly apply auricular-point-pressing with vaccaria seeds. The opposite pressing or intermittent pressing is recommended.

Basis for selection of point

Large Intestine (MA—SC4), Small Intestine (MA—SC2), Spleen (MA—IC) Stomach (MA—IC) and Sanjiao (MA—IC4) are selected to reinforce the Spleen and the Stomach and to regulate gastrointestinal function to enhance gastrointestinal peristalsis. Sympathetic (MA—AH7) is used to regulate the function of the vegetative nerve to increase intestinal peristalsis. In case of pain presenting in the incisional wound, Shenmen (MA—TF1) and Endocrine (MA—IC3) are added to relieve inflammation and cease pain.

References for treatment

Si Chengquan reported the efficacy of auricular-point-pressing on the recovery of gastrointestinal function after operation. The main points used were Stomach (MA—IC), Small Intestine (MA—SC2), Large Intestine (MA—SC4), Sanjiao (MA—IC4), Abdomen (MA—AH), Sympathetic (MA—AH7) and Endocrine (MA—IC3). Vaccaria-seed-pressing was given one day before operation and the seeds were pressed 2—3 times per day until 3 days after this operation. A total 30 cases experiencing abdominal operation were observed. Result revealed that in contrast to routine management, auricular therapy shortened the recovery time of the gastrointestinal function by 12—60 hours in 93% of the patients.

Remarks

Auricular therapy proves quite effective for postoperative abdominal distension. If it is combined with needling Zusanli (ST36), therapeutic effect can be improved.

18. Urinary calculi

Urinary calculi is a collective term for the calculi of the ureter, the Kidney, the Bladder and the urethra. When it is in the stage acute attack, severe colic suddenly develops in the lumbo-abdominal region, often radiating to the lower abdomen and external genitals and accompanied with pale complexion, cold sweating, rapid pulse, even nausea and vomiting. Red Blood cells can be found in urine examination. If infection develops, the patient will have aversion to cold, fever and pain of the kidney region. Persistent dull pain of the lumbar region may be complained by patients.

In TCM, urinary calculi belongs to the categories of *Shi Lin* (Stone Stranguria) or Xue Lin (Blood Stranguria).

Point (Fig. 5—52) and method

Main points: Kidney (MA—SC), Bladder (MA—SC8), Ureter (MA—SC7), Urethra (MA—H3), Sympathetic (MA—AH7), Sanjiao (MA—IC4).

Supplementary points: Shenmen (MA—TF1), Subcortex (MA—AT1), Ear Apex (MA—H6), Endocrine (MA—IC3).

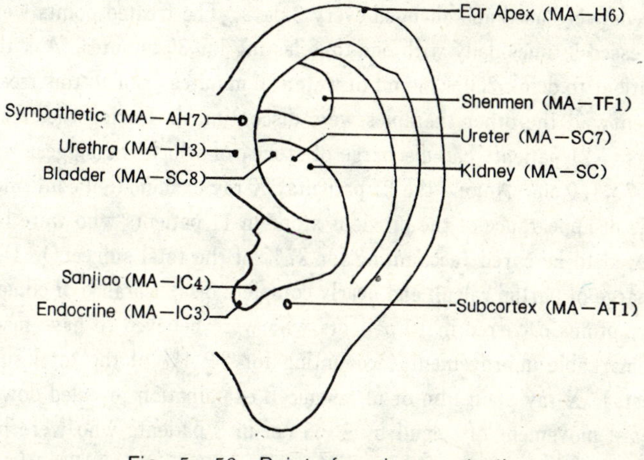

Fig. 5—52 Points for urinary calculi

Method: Mostly apply auricular-point-pressing with vaccaria seeds. The opposite pressing or intermittent pressing with strong stimulation is recommended.

Basis for selection of point

As the corresponding points to the diseased part, Kidney (MA—SC), Bladder (MA—SC8), Ureter (MA—SC7) and Urethra (MA

—H3) are selected to tonify the Kidney, to relieve stranguria and stop pain. Sanjiao (MA—IC4) is used to regulate Qi movement and clear the Water Passage. Sympathetic (MA—AH7) is employed to relieve spasm of the ureteral smooth muscle. The joint use of the above points can achieve the purpose of inducing diuresis, relieving stranguria and promoting discharge of calculi. For severe pain, Shenmen (MA—TF1) and Subcortex (MA—AT1) are added to promote the efficacy of tranquilizing the mind and ceasing pain. If fever presents due to infection, Ear Apex (MA—H6) and Endocrine (MA—IC3) are added to clear away Heat and relieve inflammation.

References for treatment

Wang Bingheng reported 41 cases of urinary calculi treated with auricular-point-pressing. Points used were Kidney (MA—SC), Bladder (MA—SC8), Ureter (MA—SC7), Urethra (MA—H3), Sanjiao (MA—IC4) and External genitals (MA—H4). Vaccaria seeds were used and changed every 3 days. The treated points were pressed 5 times daily with one time lasting for 30 minutes. Ask the patient to drink 200—250 ml of water 20 minutes prior to this treatment, all the other therapies were discontinued. During the treatment, 21 patients had discharge of stone, of which the biggest was 0.7×1.0 cm. Among the 21 patients, X-ray examination confirmed the disappearance of the previous stone in 11 patients who were believed to be cured (accounting for 27% of the total subjects). Discharge of partial calculi and nearly complete disappearance of clinical symptoms occurred in 10 patients who were believed to have made remarkable improvement (accounting for 24.4% of the total subjects). X-ray plain film or ultrasonic B examination revealed downward movement of calculi by 2—5 cm in 8 patients who were believed to have made mild improvement (accounting for 15% of the total subjects). Twelve patients did not respond (accounting for 29 of the total subjects). The total effective rate was 71%.

Wang Kemei et al reported 68 cases of urolithiasis treated with auricular-point-pressing. Points used were Kidney (MA—SC), Ureter (MA—SC7), Liver (MA—SC5), Spleen (MA—IC), Sympathetic (MA—AH7), Sanjiao (MA—IC4), Endocrine (MA—

IC3), Subcortex (MA－AT1) and Ear Apex (MA－H6). 3－5 of the above points were selected for each treatment with alternate use of the two ears. When performing treatment, first stimulate the selected points with an electrical stimulator for 20 minutes, stick then vaccaria seeds on them with plaster tape. Ask the patient to press the stuck seeds 3－4 times per day with each time lasting 10 minutes. The seeds were changed once every 3 days with 10 treatment sessions constituting one therapeutic course. Re-examination of abdominal plain film was carried out following one course of treatment. Result: cured in 20 cases, marked by complete discharge of stones which was confirmed by plain film and disappearance of symptoms; remarkable effective in 25 cases, marked by partial discharge of , reduced calculi confirmed by plain film, and obvious remission tent or disappearance of symptoms; mildly effective in 15 cases, marked by descent of stones over 5 cm and relieved symptoms; and ineffective in 8 cases. Among the 68 patients, discharge of calculi occurred in 45 patients (accounting for 60%), descent of calculi occurred in 15 cases (accounting for 22%). The total effective rate was 88%. Among the 45 patients, stone-discharge was noted one hour after treatment in 6 patients, 8 hours in 9 patients, 1－3 days in 18 patients, 4－9 days in 8 patients, and over 20 days in 4 patients. The largest stone discharged was 2.1×0.6 cm while the smallest 0.5×0.4 cm. The maximum number of the stones discharged from one patient was 5.

Remarks

Auricular-point-pressing proves quite effective for urinary calculi. The most appropriate period for treatment is the time when pain attacks, which indicates a movement of the stones. Stimulating auricular points in the active stage can elevate the rate of stone-removing as well as relieve pain.

During the treatment, ask the patient to drink more water and do moderate jumping, which will facilitate the descent and discharge of stones.

19. Postoperative and postpartum uroschesis

Uroschesis refers to fullness of the urinary bladder with urine being abnormally undischargable. If this condition develops following operation or delivery, it is called postoperative uroschesis and postpartum uroschesis, respectively. This disease is mainly manifested as fullness, distension and pain in the lower abdomen, bulge of the suprapubic region, and anuria after operation or delivery. It results from stimulation on the nerve plexus which dominates the bladder or from local edema which oppresses the bladder trigone and brings about urethral obstruction, due to operation, inhibition of micturition reflex as the result of anesthesia, or due to dysfunction of abdominal muscle to contract as the result of the incision and perineum.

In TCM, it belongs to the category of *Long Bi* (Retention of Urine).

Point (Fig. 5—53) and method

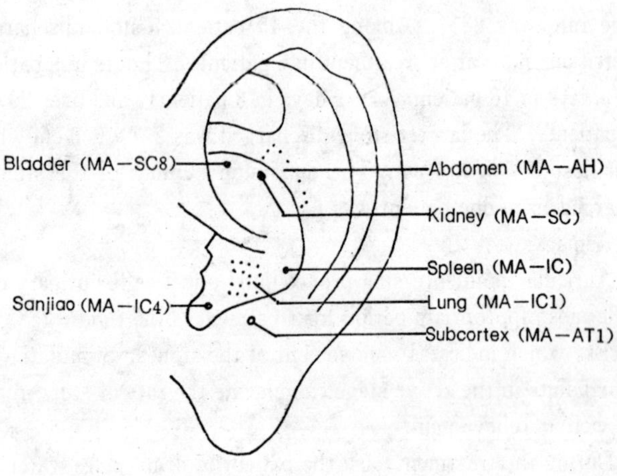

Fig. 5—53 Points for postoperative and postpartum uroschesis

Main points: Bladder (MA—SC8), Kidney (MA—SC), Sanjiao (MA—IC4).

Supplementary points: Subcortex (MA－AT1), Lung (MA－IC1), Spleen (MA－IC), Abdomen (MA－AH).

Method: Mostly apply auricular-point-pressing with vaccaria seeds. The opposite pressing or perpendicular pressing with strong stimulation is recommended.

Basis for selection of point

As the corresponding points to the diseased part, Bladder (MA－SC8) is selected to regulate the tension of the bladder and promote its contraction. Since the Kidney is exteriorly-interiorly related with the Bladder, Kidney (MA－SC) is used to tonify the Kidney Qi and strengthen the efficacy of micturition. Sanjiao (MA－IC4) is used to regulate Qi movement and clear the Water Passage. According to TCM theory, the Lung serves as the upper source of Water and dominates the dispersion and descent of Qi and the passage of Water, while the Spleen is in charge of transportation and transformation of nutrition and Water-Dampness, Lung (MA－IC1) and Spleen (MA－IC) are therefore added to regulate the Lung Qi and Spleen Qi to improve the effect of diuresis and micturition. Abdomen (MA－AH) is added to increase abdominal pressure and ameliorate the bladder contraction. Subcortex (MA－AT1) is added to regulate the cerebral cortex, to eliminate mental stress and promote the function of the bladder.

References for treatment

Chen Gongsun reported 19 cases of postoperative uroschesis treated with auricular needling at Bladder (MA－SC8), Kidney (MA－SC), Urethra (MA－H3) and Sanjiao (MA－IC4). Among the 19 patients, spontaneous micturition presented in 6 within half an hour after treatment and in 3 within 30－60 minutes. Those who did not micturate within one hour after treatment were considered ineffective.

Qiu Xiulan reported 100 cases of uroschesis due to operation on the anus treated with auricular block therapy. Use a syringe to inject 0.3－0.5 ml of 0.5%－2% of procaine or vitamin B1 injection into each of the following points to form a skin cumulus: Urethra (MA－H3), Lower section of Rectum (MA), Shenmen (MA－

TF1). Result: 97 patients micturated spontaneously within 5—20 minutes after treatment, and the rest 3 did not respond.

Ⅲ. Gynecological Diseases

1. Dysmenorrhea

Dysmenorrhea refers to pain in the lower abdomen possibly involving the lumbosacral region, which presents prior to, following or during menstruation. It can disturb the patient's work and routine life. The accompanying symptoms include nausea, vomiting, headache, dizziness, fatigue, etc. Clinically, dysmenorrhea is classified as the primary type and the secondary type. The former refers to those without organic pathological changes, it is therefore also called functional dysmenorrhea. The latter refers to those caused by organic pathological changes such as endometriosis, pelvic inflammation and submucosal myoma of the uterus.

In TCM, the same term is used. It is considered to be caused by disorder of the flow of Qi and Blood. The frequently-seen causes are emotional disturbances leading to stagnation of the Liver Qi, invasion of Cold and Dampness or overtake of cold or raw food during menstruation or after delivery, or constitutional deficiency of Yang bringing about failure to warm the uterus.

Point (Fig. 5—54) and method

Main points: Internal genitals (MA—TF), Endocrine (MA—IC3), Liver (MA—SC5), Kidney (MA—SC), Shenmen (MA—TF1), Sympathetic (MA—AH7).

Supplementary points: Stomach (MA—IC), Spleen (MA—IC), Occiput (MA—AT).

Method: Mostly apply auricular-point-pressing with vaccaria seeds. *Huo Xue Zhi Tong Gao* (Plaster for Promoting Blood Circulation and Relieving Pain) can be used for sticking the seeds. The opposite pressing or perpendicular pressing is recommended.

Basis for selection of point

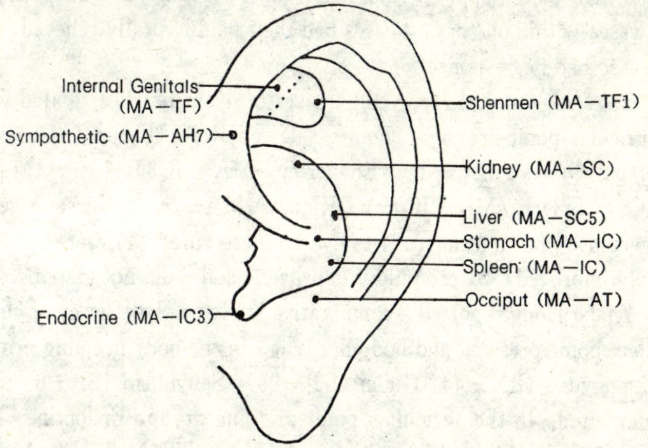

Fig. 5—54 Points for dysmenorrhea

As a corresponding point to the diseased part, Internal genitals (MA—TF) is selected to regulate Qi and Blood in the uterus. Endocrine (MA—IC3) is to regulate endocrine function. The Liver Channel curves around the external genitals and enters the lower abdomen, the Liver stores Blood, and the Kidney is the origin of the congenital constitution, according to TCM theory. Therefore, Liver (MA—SC5) and Kidney (MA—SC) are adopted to relieve the depressed Liver and tonify the Kidney Qi to regulate the Chong and Ren Channels. Shenmen (MA—TF1) and Sympathetic (MA—AH7) are for tranquilizing the mind, relieving spasm and stopping pain. Add Stomach (MA—IC) for nausea and vomiting, Occiput (MA—AT) for headache and dizziness, and Spleen (MA—IC) for fatigue due to deficiency of Qi and Blood.

References for treatment

Hong Yuhui reported 30 cases of dysmenorrhea treated with auricular- point-pressing. Points selected were Internal genitals (MA—TF), Liver (MA—SC5), Gallbladder (MA—SC6), Kidney (MA—SC), Abdomen (MA—AH), Endocrine (MA—IC3) and Adrenal Gland (MA—T). Vaccaria seeds were used for treatment and the stuck seeds were pressed over 10 times per day. Result: 18 cases had their pain stopped within half a day following the treatment and 7 cases within one day, 4 cases had their pain basically relieved, and 1 case had no response.

Dai Mingxia et al reported 85 cases of dysmenorrhea treated with auricular-point-pressing. Points selected were Uterus (MA), Adrenal Gland (MA－T), Endocrine (MA－IC3), Liver (MA－SC5), Spleen (MA－IC) and Kidney (MA－SC). Vaccaria seeds were used for treatment. Result: 59 were cured, 17 were remarkably improved, 4 were mildly improved, and 5 did not respond.

Zhang Hong reported a comparative study on the efficacy of auricular -point-pressing and body needling. In the body needling group, Guangyuan (RN－4), Guilai (ST－25), Sanyinjiao (SP－6) were punctured. In the auricular- point-pressing group, Endocrine (MA－IC3), Uterus (MA), Shenmen (MA－TF1), Liver (MA－SC5), Spleen (MA－IC) and Kidney (MA－SC) were pressed. After treatment, the effective rates of the two groups were 92% and 86%, respectively. Statistic analysis showed no significant difference between them.

Remarks

Auricular-point-pressing proves quite effective for dysmenorrhea. Clinical observation demonstrated that therapeutic effect can be improved if this treatment starts 3－5 days before menstruation. ical observation demon

2. Irregular menstruation

Irregular menstruation refers to abnormalities of menstrual cycle, quantity, color and quality. It includes preceded menstrual cycle, delayed menstrual cycle, indefinite menstrual cycle, menorrhagia and scanty menstruation.

Western medicine considers that irregular menstruation is caused by imbalance between hypothalamus, pituitary and ovary. External environment, psychic and emotional state, physical condition and other endocrine glands can affect the function of the above organs and then bring about irregular menstruation.

TCM considers that irregular menstruation is related to the Liver, the Kidney and the Spleen. It can be caused by emotional depression leading to disorder of the Liver Qi, or by deficiency of the Kidney Qi leading to failure of the Kidney in storage and discharge of Essence and debility of the Chong and Ren Channels, or by insufficiency of the Spleen Qi due to improper diet, overfatigue or anxiety.

Point (Fig. 5—55) and method

Points: Internal Genitals (MA—TF), Endocrine (MA—IC3), Subcortex (MA—AT1), Central Rim (MA—AT), Liver (MA—SC5), Spleen (MA—IC), Kidney (MA—SC).

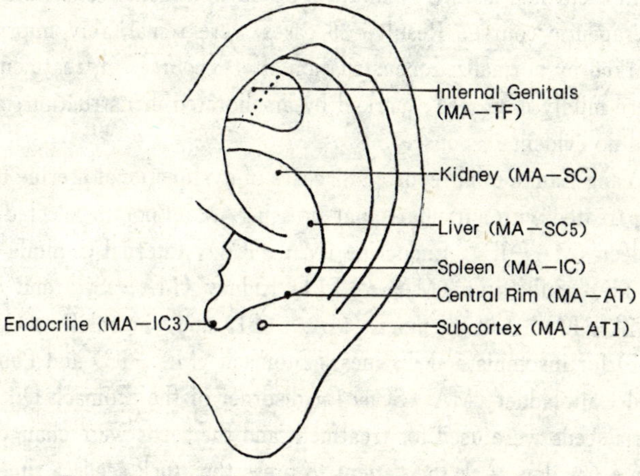

Fig. 5—55 Points for irregular menstruation

Method: Mostly apply auricular-point-pressing with vaccaria seeds. The perpendicular pressing or opposite pressing is recommended.

Basis for selection of point

As a corresponding point to the diseased part, Internal Genitals (MA—TF) is selected to regulate Qi and Blood in the uterus. Endocrine (MA—IC3), Subcortex (MA—AT1) and Central Rim (MA—AT) are used to regulate the secretary function of hypothalamus and ovary. Liver (MA—SC5) is for relieving the depressed Liver, Spleen (MA—IC) for tonifying the Spleen Qi to control Blood circulation, and Kidney (MA—SC) for regulating and replenishing the

Kidney Qi. The joint use of the above points can achieve the purpose of regulating the Chong and the Ren Channels and normalizing menstruation.

References for treatment

Zheng Ji reported 77 cases of irregular menstruation treated with auricular-point-pressing. Points selected were Shenmen (MA-TF1), Liver (MA-SC5), Kidney (MA-SC), Subcortex (MA-AT1) and Endocrine (MA-IC3). Vaccaria seeds were used for treatment and changed every 4 days with alternate use of the two ears. Ask the patient to press the stuck seeds 3-5 times per day with each time lasting 5 minutes. Seven treatments constituted one therapeutic course. Result: 25 cases were remarkably improved, marked by normalized menstruation after 3 courses of treatment; 49 were mildly improved, marked by ameliorated menstruation; and 3 had no evident response.

Yang Lanxu et al reported 82 cases of dysfunctional uterine bleeding treated with auricular-point-pressing. Main points selected were Spleen (MA-IC), Endocrine (MA-IC3), Internal Genitals (MA-TF), Subcortex (MA-AT1), Kidney (MA-SC) and Heart (MA-IC). Add Shenmen (MA-TF1) and Central Rim (MA-AT) for insomnia and dizziness, Stomach (MA-IC) and Pancreas and Gallbladder (MA-SC6) for disorder of the Stomach Qi. Vaccaria seeds were used for treatment and the seeds were changed every other day. Ask the patient to press the stuck seeds 5 times per day with each time lasting 5 minutes. Ten treatments constituted one therapeutic course. Result: 36 cases were cured (43.9%), marked by normalized menstruation; 18 were remarkably improved (20.9%), marked by nearly normal menstruation and the quantity of menses being reduced by 1/2; 16 were mildly improved (19.5%), marked by the quantity being reduced by 1/3, and 12 cases did not respond (14.6%). The total effective rate was 85.3%. Treatment sessions were 20 in the most and 5 in the least.

3. Amenorrhea

In normal condition, a female should have menses when she is about 14 years old. Amenorrhea is defined as a condition in which a female who is over 18 years old has not experienced menstruation or menstruation has ceased for more than 3 months. The former is called the primary amenorrhea while the latter the secondary amenorrhea. Amenorrhea can be caused by abnormal development of uterus or ovary, endocrine disturbance, neuropsychic factors, or some other chronic diseases. Those present in the period of pregnancy, lactation and menopause are considered to be physiological phenomenon. Amenorrhea discussed here does not include those resulting from abnormal development or organic injuries of the reproductive organs.

In TCM, this disease is also called *Bi Jing* (Amenorhea) or *Yu Shi Bu Lai* (Absence of Menstruation). It is divided as deficiency and excess types. The deficiency type is mostly caused by insufficiency of the Liver, the Kidney and the Chong Channel (Blood Sea) while the excess type is usually caused by stagnation of Qi and Blood and obstruction of Chong and Ren Channels.

Point (Fig. 5—56) and method

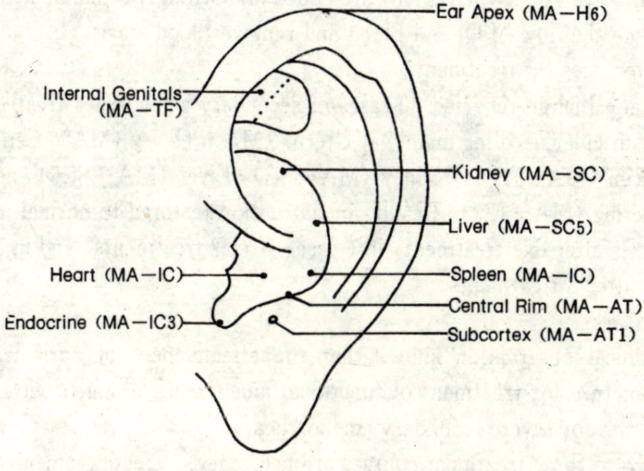

Fig. 5—56 Points for amenorrhea

Main points: Internal Genitals (MA—TF), Endocrine (MA—IC3), Subcortex (MA—AT1), Central Rim (MA—AT).

Supplementary points: Liver (MA—SC5), Spleen (MA—IC), Kidney (MA—SC), Heart (MA—IC), Ear Apex (MA—H6).

Method: Mostly apply auricular-point-pressing with vaccaria seeds. For the excess type, *Xiang Gui Huo Xue Gao* (Plaster for Promoting Blood Circulation Mainly with Moschus and Cortex Cinnamomi) can be used for sticking the seeds. The intermittent pressing is recommended for the deficiency type while the perpendicular pressing or opposite pressing for the excess type.

Basis for selection of point

As a corresponding point to the diseased part, Internal Genitals (MA—TF) is selected to regulate Qi and Blood in the uterus. Endocrine (MA—IC3), Subcortex (MA—AT1) and Central Rim (MA—AT) are selected on the basis of Western medicine to regulate the function of endocrine and ovary. According to TCM syndrome identification, for the deficiency type, Liver (MA—SC5), Spleen (MA—IC) and Kidney (MA—SC) are added to replenish their corresponding viscera, to invigorate Qi and enrich Blood, while for the excess type, Liver (MA—SC5), Spleen (MA—IC), Heart (MA—IC) and Ear Apex (MA—H6) are added and strongly stimulated to promote the flow of Qi and Blood and remove Blood stasis.

References for treatment

Huang Lichun reported 20 cases of secondary amenorrhea treated with auricular needling mainly at Uterus (MA), Ovary (MA), Central Rim (MA—AT), Kidney (MA—SC), Liver (MA—SC5) and Endocrine (MA—IC3). Result: menstruation restored to normal in 12 cases after one treatment, in 6 cases after 2 treatments, and in 3 cases after 3 treatments.

Remarks

Clinical observation shows that the effectiveness of auricular acupuncture for treatment of functional amenorrhea is much better than that for severe secondary amenorrhea.

Two to three treatment courses are necessary in treating amenorrhea with auricular acupuncture. Patients who have restored their menstruation following one treatment course still need to continue this treatment until the efficacy is maintained or menstrual cycle is normalized.

4. Climacteric syndrome

Climacteric syndrome is caused by dysfunction of the endocrine and vegetative nerve due to decline of the ovary in climacteric females. It is manifested as irregular menstruation, palpitation, irritability, feverish sensation in the chest, palms and soles, flushed face, perspiration, or edema, loose stools, soreness and weakness of the lumbar region and legs, even hypochondriac delusion and emotional disturbance.

In TCM, climacteric syndrome is believed to be caused by decline of the Kidney Qi, deficiency of the Chong and Ren Channels, depletion of the Tian Gui (Reproductive Essence), and insufficiency of Essence and Blood, leading to failure of the Kidney Yin in nourishing the Liver Yang and imbalance between Yin and Yang.

Point (Fig. 5—57) and method

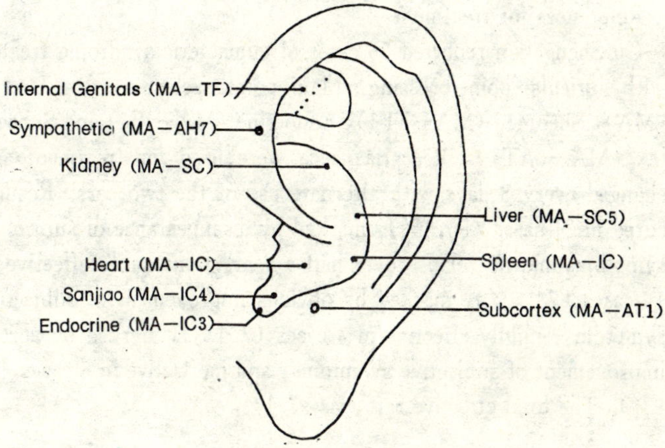

Fig. 5—57 Points for climacteric synerome

Main points: Internal Genitals (MA—TF), Subcortex (MA—AT1), Endocrine (MA—IC3), Liver (MA—SC5), Kidney (MA—SC).

Supplementary points: Heart (MA — IC), Shenmen (MA —

TF1), Sympathetic (MA—AH7), Spleen (MA—IC), Sanjiao (MA—IC4).

Method: Mostly apply auricular-point-pressing with vaccaria seeds or *Xiao Yao Wan* (Easy Pill). The intermittent pressing with strong stimulation is recommended.

Basis for selection of point

Internal Genitals (MA—TF) is selected as a corresponding point to the diseased part. Endocrine (MA—IC3) and Subcortex (MA—AT1) are employed to regulate the function of endocrine and ovary. Liver (MA—SC5) and Kidney (MA—SC) are used to replenish the Kidney (Water) for nourishing the Liver (Wood), to strengthen the Chong and Ren Channels and regulate Yin and Yang. Add Heart (MA—IC) and Shenmen (MA—TF1) to tranquilize and calm the mind for palpitation, irritability and insomnia, Sympathetic (MA—AH7) to regulate vegetative nerve for flushed face and profuse perspiration, and Spleen (MA—IC) and Sanjiao (MA—IC4) to replenish the Spleen and eliminate Dampness for edema.

References for treatment

Gu Shengchun reported 56 cases of climacteric syndrome treated with auricular-point-pressing. Main points selected were Uterus (MA), Shenmen (MA—TF1), Endocrine (MA—IC3) and Subcortex (MA—AT1). Vaccaria seeds were used for treatment and changed every 3 days with alternate use of the two ears. Result: cured in 31 cases (55,4%), marked by disappearance of subjective symptoms and no relapse over half a year; remarkably effective in 16 cases (28. 6%), marked by obvious improvement of subjective symptoms; mildly effective in 4 cases (7. 1%), marked by partial improvement of subjective symptoms; and ineffective in 5 cases (8. 9%). The total effective rate was 91. 1%.

5. Premenstrual syndrome

Premenstrual syndrome refers to one or several physiologic, psychic or behavior changes before menstruation. Its clinical manifestations may be irritability, depression, headache, dizziness, insomnia, distending pain in breast, abdominal distension with sinking sensation and edema. Those symptoms present periodically, i. e., worsening during the period of menstruation but disappearing immediately after it.

The etiology of this disease is unclear and supposed to be related with periodic imbalance of sexual hormones and psychic factors.

In TCM, there is no corresponding term for this disease. According to the symptoms presented before and during menstruation, it can be attributed to the categories of emotional disturbance during menstruation, headache during menstruation, edema during menstruation and distending pain in breast during menstruation. The common causes of this disease are dysfunction of Zang-Fu organs, stagnation of the Liver Qi and deficiency of the Liver Yin and the Kidney Yin.

Point (Fig. 5—58) and method

Main points: Internal Genitals (MA—TF), Liver (MA—SC5), Kidney (MA—SC), Sympathetic (MA—AH7), Subcortex (MA—AT1).

Supplementary points: Heart (MA—IC), Shenmen (MA—TF1), Spleen (MA—IC), Sanjiao (MA—IC4), Chest (MA—AH11).

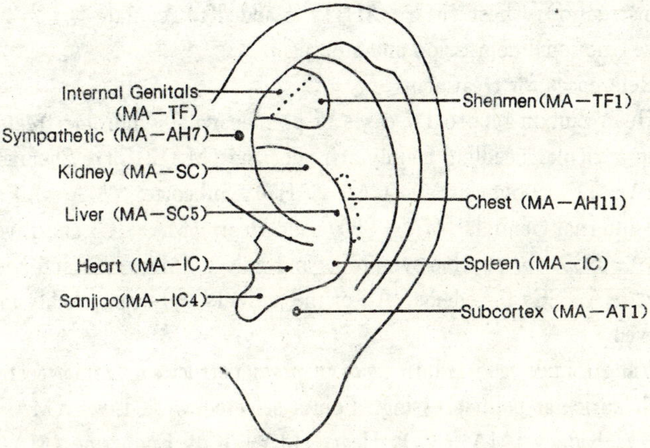

Fig. 5—58 Points for premenstrual syndrome

Method: Mostly apply auricular-point-pressing with vaccaria seeds. The perpendicular pressing or intermittent pressing is recommended.

Basis for selection of point

According to TCM theory, this disease should be treated based on the therapeutic principle of regulating the function of the Zang-Fu organs. Internal Genitals (MA—TF), Liver (MA—SC5) and Kidney (MA—SC) are selected to tonify the Kidney and replenish Essence, to soothe the depressed Liver and regulate Qi, and to relieve emotional depression. According to Western medicine, Sympathetic (MA—AH7) and Subcortex (MA—AT1) are used to regulate endocrine and vegetative nerve to restore the coordination of hormones. For emotional disturbances during menstruation, Heart (MA—IC) and Shenmen (MA—TF1) are added to calm the Heart and tranquilize the mind. For headache and dizziness during menstruation, Occiput (MA—AT) and Forehead (MA—AT) are added to tranquilize the mind, to stop pain, to calm Wind and to relieve dizziness. For edema during menstruation, Spleen (MA—IC) and Sanjiao (MA—IC4) are added to reinforce the Spleen, to eliminate Dampness and clear the Sanjiao. For distending pain in breast during menstruation, Chest (MA—AH11) is added to regulate Qi, to relieve emotional depression and stop pain.

References for treatment

Guan Zunxin reported 7 cases of premenstrual syndrome treated with auricular needling mainly at Endocrine (MA—IC3), Shenmen (MA—TF1), Sympathetic (MA—AH7), Subcortex (MA—AT1) and Internal Genitals (MA—TF). Add Heart (MA—IC) and Liver (MA—SC5) for psychic symptoms and Spleen (MA—IC) and Kidney (MA—SC) for edema. All of the patients were remarkably improved.

Yang Lanxu reported 15 cases of premenstrual syndrome treated with auricular-point-pressing. Points selected were Liver (MA—SC5), Kidney (MA—SC), Heart (MA—IC), Endocrine (MA—IC3), Internal Genitals (MA—TF), Sympathetic (MA—AH7), Subcortex (MA—AT1) and Shenmen (MA—TF1). Treatment with vaccaria seeds was carried out 5 days prior to menstruation. Result: 9 cases were cured and 6 cases were remarkably improved.

6. Malposition of fetus

Malposition of fetus refers to an over 30 weeks' fetus in an abnormal position of the uterus. It is mostly seen in multiparas or those with loose abdominal wall. Malposition of fetus is asympomatic and can only be found through prenatal examination. Except occipitoanterior position, all the other positions are abnormal and may result in difficult labor.

In TCM, the same term is used.

Point (Fig. 5—59) and method

Points: Internal Genitals (MA—TF), Abdomen (MA—AH), Sympathetic (MA—AH7), Subcortex (MA—AT1), Liver (MA—SC5), Spleen (MA—IC), Kidney (MA—SC).

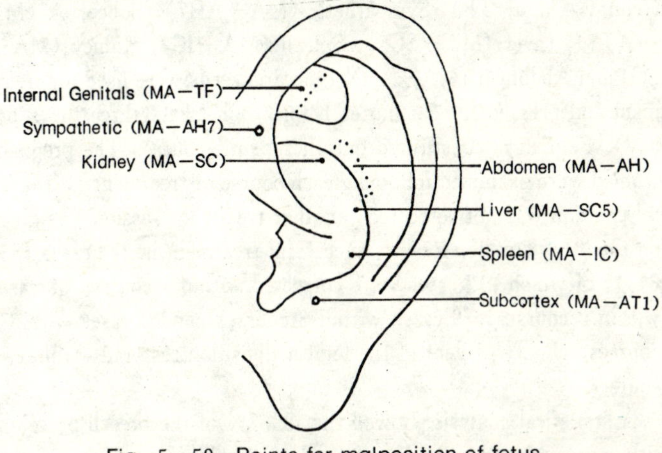

Fig. 5—59 Points for malposition of fetus

Method: Mostly apply auricular-point-pressing with vaccaria seeds. The intermittent pressing with weak stimulation is recommended.

Basis for selection of point

Internal Genitals (MA—TF) is selected to regulate Qi and Blood to nourish the uterus. Abdomen (MA—AH) has the function of regulating the abdominal muscle to maintain its normal tension. Since the uterus is controlled by the vegetative nerve, Sympathetic (MA—AH7) and Subcortex (MA—AT1) are employed to regulate the functions of the cerebral cortex and vegetative nerve. According to TCM theory, Liver (MA—SC5), Spleen (MA—IC) and Kidney (MA—SC) are used to replenish the Liver and the Kidney and regulate Qi and Blood to nourish the fetus. The joint use of the above points can activate the fetal movement and strengthen the physiological uterine contraction to facilitate the correction of fetal position.

References for treatment

Qing Guangfeng reported 413 cases of malposition of fetus treated with auricular-point-pressing therapy. Among them, 323 were primiparae and the remaining 90 cases were pluriparae. There were 386 cases of breech presentation, 25 cases of horizontal presentation and 2 cases of footling presentation. Points selected were Internal Genitals (MA—TF), Sympathetic (MA—AH7), Subcortex (MA—AT1), Liver (MA—SC5), Spleen (MA—IC), Kidney (MA—SC) and Abdomen (MA—AH). Vaccaria seeds were used for treatment and pressed for 5 minutes before each meal (three times per day). Four days constituted one therapeutic course. The pregnant women were examined following each course of treatment. If the fetal position was not corrected, another treatment session was given on the other auricle. Result: successful treatment in 344 cases (83.3%), of which 212 cases were corrected within 1 course, 99 cases within 2 courses, 29 cases within 3 courses, and 4 cases within 4 courses. Ninety percent of the fetal malposition restored within two courses.

A statistical analysis showed that 82.2% of the breech presentation was corrected and 84% of the horizontal presentation was corrected. Both cases of footling presentation were corrected. There was no significant difference between different malpositions of fetus ($P<0.05$). For the 212 cases in pregnancy between 30—33 weeks, the successful rate of correcting fetal position was 91%. For the 125 cases in pregnancy between 33—37 weeks, the successful rate was 80.6%. For the 37 cases in pregnancy over 37 weeks, the successful rate was 47.1%. The result indicated that the shorter the pregnant period, the higher the corrective rate ($P<0.01$).

7. Leukorrhagia

Physiologically, there is a little amount of mucous or white secretary liquid in the vagina for moistening the genital epithelia, which is called leukorrhea. Leukorrhagia refers to continuous and abnormal increase of the yellowish or red-white leukorrhea with dilute or purulent quality and foul odor. It is mostly caused by inflammation or tumor of the genitals.

In TCM, the same term is used. It is considered to be caused by deficiency of the Spleen and Kidney and downward flow of Dampness-Heat leading to poor restriction of the Dai Channel and the Ren Channel.

Point (Fig. 5—60) and method

Points: Internal Genitals (MA—TF), Pelvis (MA—TF), Endocrine (MA—IC3), Adrenal Gland (MA—T).

Supplementary points: Spleen (MA—IC), Lung (MA—IC1), Kidney (MA—SC), Liver (MA—SC5), Sanjiao (MA—IC4), External Genitals (MA—H4).

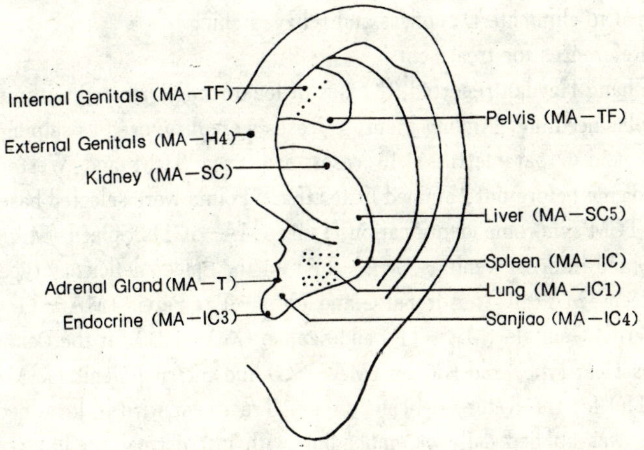

Fig. 5—60 Points for leukorrhagia

Method: Mostly apply auricular-point-pressing with vaccaria seeds. The perpendicular pressing or intermittent pressing is recommended.

Basis for selection of point

As the corresponding points to the diseased part, Internal Genitals (MA—TF) and Pelvis (MA—TF) are selected in combination with Endocrine (MA—IC3) and Adrenal Gland (MA—T) to dredge Channels and Collaterals, to relieve inflammation and cease leukorrhagia. If profuse white leukorrhea is accompanied with poor appetite, loose stools or diarrhea and pale tongue with white and greasy coating, which is differentiated as deficiency of the Spleen, Spleen (MA—IC) and Lung (MA—IC1) are added to invigorate the Spleen and eliminate Dampness. If leukorrhea is white and thin accompanied with soreness of the lumbar region, lassitude, frequent urination, pale tongue with white coating, which is differentiated as deficiency of the Kidney, Kidney (MA—SC) should be added to tonify the Kidney Qi. If leukorrhea is yellow with foul odor and accompanied with scanty dark urine, Liver (MA—SC5) and Sanjiao (MA—IC4) should be added to clear away Dampness-Heat from the Liver and remove Toxic Materials. If leukorrhea is accompanied with pruritus of the vulva, External Genitals (MA—H4) should be added to eliminate Dampness and relieve itching.

References for treatment

Zhang Heyuan reported 21 cases of leukorrhagia treated with auricular needling. Among them, 15 cases were diagnosed as salpingitis, and 6 parametritis; 13 cases had tried TCM and Western medicine before but obtained little effect. Points were selected based on TCM syndrome identification: Lung (MA—IC1), Spleen (MA—IC) and Internal Genitals (MA—TF) for the Spleen deficiency type; Spleen (MA—IC), Adrenal Gland (MA—T), Pelvis (MA—TF), Internal Genitals (MA—TF) and Sanjiao (MA—IC4) for the Dampness-Heat type; and Kidney (MA—SC) and Internal Genitals (MA—TF) for the Kidney deficiency type. Treatment with filiform needles was applied daily or embedding with intradermal needles was applied every 3 days. Result: cured in 20 cases, marked by normal leukorrhea and disappearance of accompanying symptoms; and unclear result in 1 case for the patient did not return after first embedding of intradermal needles.

Remarks

Since leukorrhagia is only a clinical symptom, it is necessary to find out the causes and make a definite diagnosis before treatment. If a patient presents constant leukorrhea with reddish and white discharge, carcinoma should be excluded at first.

8. Postpartum agalactosia

Postpartum agalactosia refers to inadequate lactation of milk that is not enough to meet the need of a baby. Except a few cases resulting from hypoplasia of the breast, most are caused by malnutrition of the body, dysfunction of the vegetative nerve, psychic stimulation, or emotional depression.

In TCM, postpartum agalactosia is classified as the deficiency type and the excess type. Those resulting from weakness of the body and deficiency of Qi and Blood that bring about lack of source to produce milk are identified as the deficiency type, which is manifested as no distending sensation in the breast and a little lactation of milk 48 hours after delivery. Those resulting from emotional stimulation that leads to disorder of Qi, incoordination between Qi and Blood and blockage of Channels are identified as the excess type, which is manifested as distending pain of the breast and absence of milk lactation.

Point (Fig. 5—61) and method

Main points: Chest (MA—AH11), Endocrine (MA—IC3), Sympathetic (MA—AH7).

Supplementary points: Spleen (MA—IC), Stomach (MA—IC), Liver (MA—SC5).

Method: Mostly apply auricular-point-pressing with vaccaria seeds. The intermittent pressing with weak force is recommended for the deficiency type while the perpendicular pressing or opposite pressing for the excess type.

Basis for selection of point

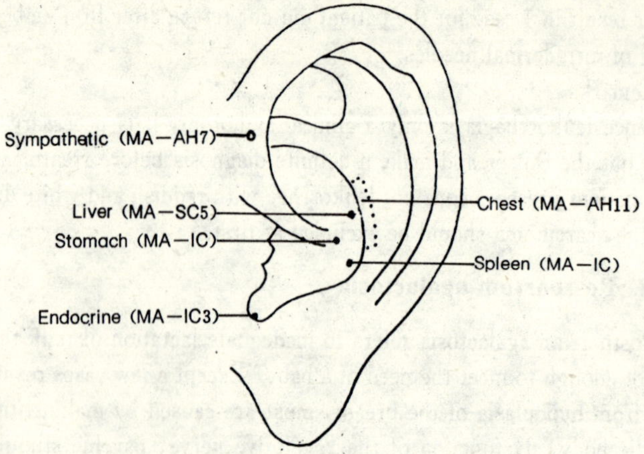

Fig. 5—61 Points for postpartum agalactosia

Chest (MA—AH11) is adopted to promote the flow of Qi and Blood in the local area. Endocrine (MA—IC3) and Sympathetic (MA—AT1) are selected to regulate the endocrine and vegetative nerve function to promote milk lactation. For the deficiency type, Spleen (MA—IC) and Stomach (MA—IC) are added to reinforce the Spleen and the Stomach to enrich the source of Qi and Blood. For the excess type, Liver (MA—SC5) is added to relieve the depressed Liver, to regulate the movement of Qi, to ease the mind, to dredge Channels and remove Blood stasis.

References for treatment

Jing Yanzu reported 126 cases of short-term hypogalactia treated with auricular needling. One to two treatments can restore lactation of milk to normal. As to those with long-term hypogalactia (over one month), this treatment can increase lactation but the milk may not be enough to meet the need of a baby.

Remarks

Auricular therapy proves quite effective for short-term hypogalactia. However, it is not obviously effective for the treatment of hypogalactia with a long-term duration or for that due to mammary hypoplasia.

Ⅳ. Diseases of the Eye, Ear, Nose, Throat and Mouth Cavity

1. Toothache

Toothache, as a common symptom in oral diseases, can be caused by disease of the teeth, periodontal tissues, jaw bone or nerves. It may also be a reaction of a general disease. The common causes are dental caries, pulpitis, epical periodonitis, pericoronitis and periodonitis. Toothache are often aggravated by stimulation of cold, hot, sour and sweet.

In TCM, toothache is basically divided as deficiency Fire type and excess Fire type. Those that result from deficiency of the Kidney Yin leading to hyperactivity of the deficient Fire are identified as the deficiency Fire toothache. It is manifested as intermittent dull pain which is better during day time but worse at night, accompanied with loose teeth, soreness of lumbar region, lassitude and fatigue. Those that result from retention of Heat in the Large Intestine and Stomach or invasion of Wind resulting in Fire in the Yangming Channel are identified as the excess Fire toothache. It is manifested as severe pain accompanied with swollen gum, foul mouth and constipation.

Point (Fig. 5—62) and method

Main points: Teeth (MA—L), Jam (MA—L), Anterior Ear Lobe (MA—L), Endocrine (MA—IC3), Subcortex (MA—AT1), Shenmen (MA—TF1).

Supplementary points: Stomach (MA—IC), Large Intestine (MA SC4), Kidney (MA—SC).

Method: Mostly apply auricular-point-pressing with vaccaria seeds. The opposite pressing or the perpendicular pressing is recommended.

Basis for selection of point

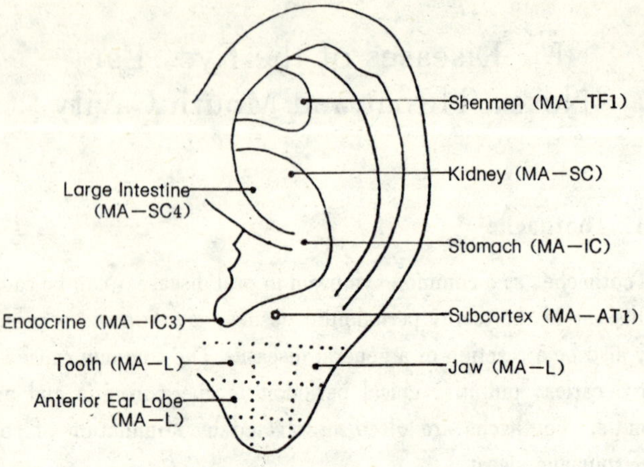

Fig. 5—62 Points for toothache

Tooth (MA—L) and Jaw (MA—L) are selected as the corresponding points to the diseased part. Anterior Ear Lobe (MA—L), also called "anesthetic point for tooth extraction," is an empirical point for toothache. Endocrine (MA—IC3), Subcortex (MA—AT1) and Shenmen (MA—TF1) are selected to relieve inflammation, to tranquilize the mind and stop pain. For the excess Fire type, Stomach (MA—IC) and Large Intestine (MA—SC4) are added to clear away the Yangming Heat to enhance the efficacy of relieving inflammation and pain. For the deficiency Fire type, Kidney (MA—SC) is added to reduce Fire by nourishing the Kidney Yin, thus relieving pain.

References for treatment

Han Biying reported 72 cases of toothache treated by pressing positive reaction spots with a probe. Method: on the interior side of the antitragus, draw an equilateral triangle based on the line connecting Apex of Antitragus (MA—AT) with Central Rim (MA—AT). Detect a positive spot with a probe in the triangle, such as angioplerosis, patch aula or spotty pimple, press it slightly for a while to produce a sharp stabbing pain, then press heavily towards the rim of antitragus to produce an intolerable pain. Generally, the toothache will be relieved simultaneously. Result: 69 cases were cured, accounting for 95.85% of the total. Comparing with a routine acupuncture group (n=51, the cure rate being 78.51%), there was significant difference ($P<0.05$) in favor of the auricular therapy.

Zhou Li reported 30 cases of toothache treated by auricular acupuncture at Sanjiao (MA—IC4) with a probe. Method: first detect a tenderness in the point locus, then puncture it with a filiform needle after sterilization. Treatment was performed once per day with 4 treatments constituting one course. For those afraid of needling, auricular-point-pressing with vaccaria seeds can be applied. Ask the patient to press the stuck seeds until a hot sensation was produced. Four days constituted one therapeutic course. Of the 30 cases, 23 accepted needling and 7 auricular pressing. Result: in the needling group, after 1—4 treatments, 16 were cured, 6 were improved, and 1 did not respond; in the auricular pressing group, after one course of treatment, 5 were cured and 2 were improved.

2. Recurrent ulcerative stomatitis

Recurrent ulcerative stomatitis, also called recurrent aphthous stomatitis, or recurrent ulcer of the mouth, is characterized by periodic or irregular recurrent ulceration of the oral mucosa and subsequent pain. The severity of the manifestations varies with the pathological changes of the disease. In the early stage of a mild case, there may present congestion, edema and maliary vesicle in the local mucusa and a sensation of tightness, burning or slight pain. When ulceration is formed, there will present circular or elliptical ulcer several millimeters in diameter with depressed surface and slightly prominent margin, and the patient feels a sensation of burning pain which is aggravated by eating or stimulation of sour, saltiness or pungency. In severe cases, there may present more and bigger ulceration and more severe pain, accompanied with salivation and inconvenience in speaking, drinking and eating. Some patients may have fever, headache, sore throat, submaxillary lymphadenectasis, dry mouth and constipation. In Western medicine, the cause of this disease remains unclear. However, recent developments of immunological theory show that it is associated with autoimmunity.

In TCM, this disease belongs to the categories of Kou Chuang (Aphthac), Kou Yang (Mouth Sore) and Kou Gan (Aphthac in Children). It is classified into the deficiency type and the excess type. The excess type is mostly caused by accumulated Heat in the Heart and Spleen or invasion of exogenous Heat while the deficiency type is frequently caused by hyperactivity of Fire and flaring up of Yang resulting from Yin deficiency.

Point (Fig. 5—63) and method

Main points: Mouth (MA—IC5), Tongue (MA—L), Shenmen (MA—TF1), Subcortex (MA—AT1), Endocrine (MA—IC3).

Supplementary points: Heart (MA—IC), Small Intestine (MA—SC2), Spleen (MA—IC), Kidney (MA—SC), Sympathetic (MA—AH7).

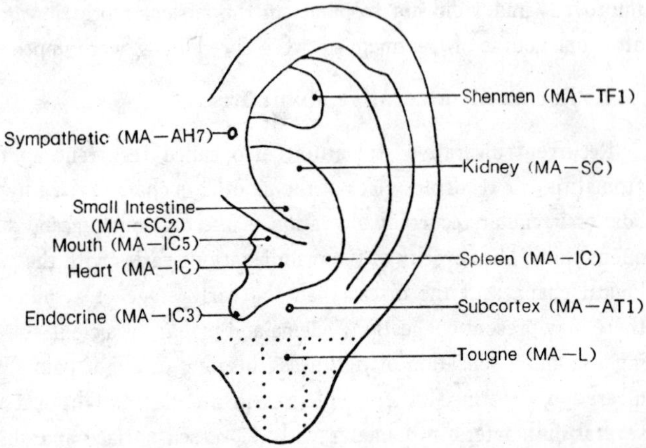

Fig. 5—63 Points for recurrent ulcerative stomatitis

Method: Mostly apply auricular-point-pressing with vaccaria seeds or *Bing Pian* (Borneolum Syntheticum). The opposite pressing or the intermittent pressing is recommended.

Basis for selection of point

As the corresponding points to the diseased part, Mouth (MA—IC5) and Tongue (MA—L) are selected to relieve inflammation and pain. According to Western medicine, Shenmen (MA—TF1), Subcortex (MA—AT1) and Endocrine (MA—IC3) are used to improve the efficacy of relieving inflammation, swelling and pain, regulating endocrine to enhance the immunological function, thus promoting recovery of ulceration. For those due to accumulated Heat in the Heart and Spleen, Heart (MA—IC), Small Intestine (MA—SC2) and Spleen (MA—IC) are added to clear away Heat, to replenish the Spleen and eliminate Dampness. For those due to invasion of exogenous Heat, Ear Apex (MA—H6) is added to clear away Heat. And for those due to hyperactivity of the deficiency Fire, Kidney (MA—SC), Heart (MA—IC) and Sympathetic (MA—AH7) are added to nourish the Kidney and purge the Fire.

References for treatment

Sun Zhenyu reported 60 cases of ulcerative stomatitis. Points selected were: Mouth (MA—IC5), Lung (MA—IC1) and Subcortex (MA—AT1) as main points, Heart (MA—IC), Large Intestine (MA—IC4), Small Intestine (MA—IC2), Spleen (MA—IC) and Shenmen (MA—TF1) as supplementary points. *Mu Xiang Shun Qi Wan* was used to press the points bilaterally. The pills were changed every other day with 5 treatments constituting one therapeutic course. Result: cured in 53 cases (88.3%), marked by healing of ulcer and no pain or burning sensation when eating and drinking; improved in 6 cases (10%), marked by shrunk ulcer, reduced redness and swelling and obviously improved subjective symptoms; ineffective in 1 case (1.7%), marked by no obvious improvement of symptoms and signs after 5 treatments. The total effective rate was 98.3%. Forty-nine patients were cured within 2 treatments, accounting for 81.67 % of the total subjects. The author considered that although ulcerative stomatitis has a tendency towards spontaneous cure, the short treatment course and obvious improvement can confirm the efficacy of auricular therapy.

Wang Jun reported 100 cases of recurrent ulcerative stomatitis. Of them, the longest disease history was 15 years while the shortest 2 years. Shenmen (MA—TF1), Mouth (MA—IC5) and Tongue (MA—L) were employed as main points. Supplementary points were added according to syndrome identification: Sympathetic (MA—AH7) for type of Seasonal Toxin; Heart (MA—IC), Liver (MA—SC5) and Small Intestine (MA—SC2) for type of Liver Fire; Liver (MA—SC5), Spleen (MA—IC), Stomach (MA—IC) and Large Intestine (MA—SC4) for type of stagnation of the Liver Qi and deficiency of the Spleen; Heart (MA—IC), Kidney (MA—SC), Sympathetic (MA—AH7) and Adrenal Gland (MA—T) for deficiency of the Heart Yin and the Kidney Yin; Endocrine (MA—IC3) and Internal Genitals (MA—TF) for female patients. Filiform needles were used to puncture the selected points and retained for 30 minutes during each treatment. Treatment was given once per day with 5 treatments constituting one therapeutic course. Result: cured in 57 cases, marked by healing of ulcer and no relapse within half a year; remarkably improved in 33 cases, marked by healing of ulcer and no relapse within three months; and improved in 10 cases, marked by healing of ulcer and no relapse within one month. The total effective rate was 100%.

3. Tonsillitis

Tonsillitis refers to the inflammation of the tonsil. Based on different nature of inflammation, it is divided into two types: acute tonsillitis and chronic tonsillitis. The acute tonsillitis is a kind of nonspecific inflammation, frequently occurring in young people aged between 10—30 years in spring and autumn. The chronic tonsillitis mostly results from recurrent attack of the acute one, frequently encountered in people aged between 7—14 years.

The acute tonsillitis is characterized by pain and congestion of throat and swollen tonsil covered with yellowish white exudate, accompanied with fever, headache, mandibular lymphadenectasis, etc. The chronic tonsillitis is characterized as discomfort sensation of throat, headache, weakness of four limbs and nocturnal low fever, chronic congestive tonsil with dark red or purple color and uneven surface, and enlarged lymph nodes possibly felt at the angle of mandible on both sides.

In TCM, tonsillitis belongs to the category of *Ru E* (Throat

Moth). Acute tonsillitis is called *Feng Re Ru E* (Wind-Heat Throat Moth) while the chronic one is called *Yin Xu Ru E* (Yin Deficiency Throat Moth). It is considered to be caused by invasion of Wind-Heat or upwards steaming of the Fire in the Lung and the Stomach.

Point (Fig. 5—64) and method

Main points: Ear Apex (MA—H6), Tonsil (MA—L), Pharynx and Larynx (MA—T3), Lung (MA—IC1), Stomach (MA—IC), Endocrine (MA—IC3), Adrenal Gland (MA—T).

Supplementary points: Helix 1—3 (MA—H), Helix 4—6 (MA—H), Kidney (MA—SC).

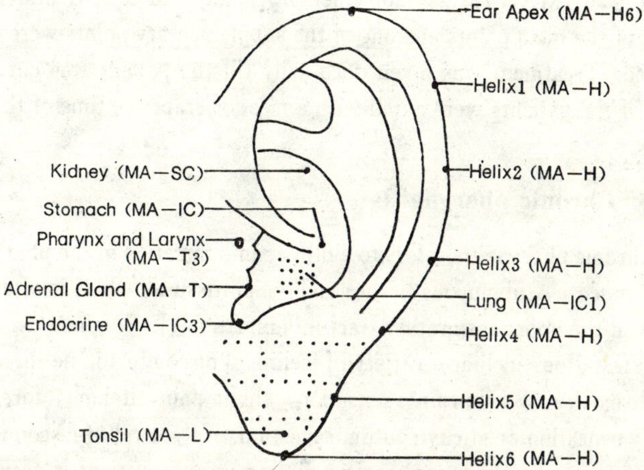

Fig. 5—64 Points for tonsillitis

Method: Mostly apply auricular-point-pressing with vaccaria seeds. For acute tonsillitis, Ear Apex (MA—H6) should be pricked to cause bleeding. The opposite pressing or perpendicular pressing is recommended.

Basis for selection of point

Ear Apex (MA—H6) is selected to clear away Heat and Toxic Materials. As the corresponding points to the diseased part, Tonsil (MA—L) and Pharynx and Larynx (MA—T3) are used to relieve sore throat and subdue swelling. Lung (MA—IC1) and Stomach (MA—IC) are selected to clear away Heat from the Lung and the

Stomach to fresh the throat. Endocrine (MA—IC3) and Adrenal Gland (MA—AT) are used to clear away Heat, to relieve inflammation and subdue swelling. For acute tonsillitis, Helix 1—3 (MA—H) are added to promote the efficacy of clearing away Heat and eliminating Toxic Materials. For chronic tonsillitis, Helix 1—3 (MA—H) and Kidney (MA—SC) are added to nourish Yin and clear away Heat.

References for treatment

A report of 25 cases of acute tonsillitis treated with auricular needling. Helix 6,4,3 (MA—H) were taken as main points and Helix 1,2,5 (MA—H) as supplementary points. In each treatment, two of the main points and one of the supplementary points were selected. Treatment was given once daily till the patient was cured. All of the patients were cured with a mean therapeutic time of three days.

4. Chronic pharyngitis

Chronic pharyngitis refers to a diffuse inflammation in the pharyngeal mucosa, submucous tissues and lymph tissues, which is often a part of the upper respiratory tract inflammation. Its common clinical manifestations include a variety of feeling of discomfort in he throat, such as dryness, burning sensation, slight pain, itching, foreign body sensation or sticky sputum sensation. To get rid of discomfort of the throat in the morning after getting up, the patient is used to coughing to expectorate sticky sputum, possibly accompanied with vomiting. Examination shows chronic congestion and thickening of the pharyngeal mucosa, enlargement of lymph follicle, and/or atrophy and thinning of pharyngeal mucosa.

In TCM, chronic pharyngitis belongs to the categories of *Xu Huo Hou Bi* (Sore Throat of Deficiency Fire) or *Yin Xu Hou Bi* (Sore Throat of Yin Deficiency). It is considered to be caused by constitutional deficiency of the Lung and the Kidney or protracted Wind-Heat sore throat which results in impairment of the Liver and the Kidney and insufficiency of Body Fluid leading to failure of nourishment of the Channels of the throat and flaming-up of the deficiency

Fire along Channels to the throat.

Point (Fig. 5—65) and method

Main points: Pharynx and Larynx (MA—T3), Mouth (MA—IC5), Lung (MA—IC1), Kidney (MA—SC), Endocrine (MA—IC3), Adrenal Gland (MA—T).

Supplementary points: Sanjiao (MA—IC4), Ear Apex (MA—H6).

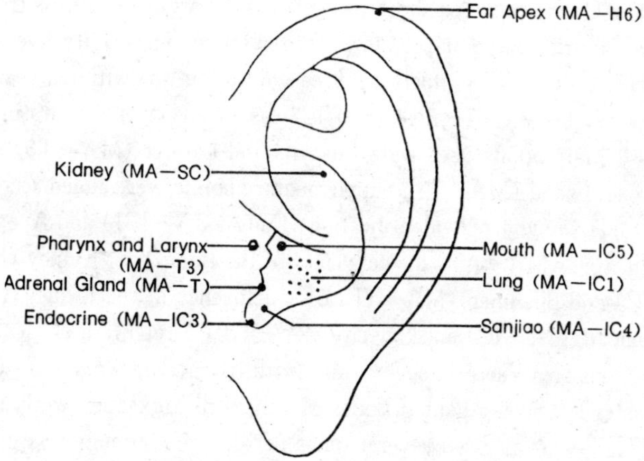

Fig. 5—65 Points for chronic pharyngitis

Method: Mostly apply auricular-point-pressing with vaccaria seeds, *Liu Shen Wan* (Six Miraculous Drugs Pill), *Yan Hou Wan* (Relieving Sore Throat Pill) or *Bing Pian* (Borneol). The perpendicular pressing or intermittent pressing is recommended.

Basis for selection of point

This disease should be treated with the therapeutic principle of nourishing Yin and clearing away Heat to relieve sore throat. As the corresponding points to the diseased part, Pharynx and Larynx (MA—T3) and Mouth (MA—IC5) are selected to subdue swelling and fresh the throat. Throat serves as the door of the Lung, Lung (MA—IC1) is therefore used to clear away Heat from the Lung. Kidney (MA—SC) is combined with Lung (MA—IC1) to nourish Yin of the Lung and the Kidney. Endocrine (MA—IC3) and Adrenal Gland (MA－T) are adopted to relieve inflammation and swelling to improve the efficacy of the above points in clearing away Heat and relieving sore throat. In case of severe dry and sore throat accompanied with constipation, Sanjiao (MA－IC4) and Ear Apex (MA－H6) are added to strengthen the effect of clearing away Heat and purging Fire.

References for treatment

Ding Quang reported short-term effects of chronic tonsillitis treated with auricular-point-pressing. Two hundred and seventy-five cases were observed, of which the disease duration was within 1 year in 72 cases, between 2－5 years in 122 cases, and over 5 years in 81 cases. Main points used were Pharynx and Larynx (MA－T3) and Adrenal Gland (MA－T). Supplementary points were added according to TCM syndrome identification: Lung (MA－IC1) and Apex of Antitragus (MA－AT) for deficiency of the Lung Yin, Kidney (MA－SC) and Shenmen (MA－TF1) for deficiency of the Kidney Yin, Stomach (MA－IC) and Spleen (MA－IC) for retention of Heat in the Stomach. Vaccaria seeds stuck with *She Xiang Zhang Gu Gao* (Plaster for Strengthening Bones Mainly with Moxchus) were used and they were pressed several times per day. Treatment was given every other day with 10 treatments constituting one therapeutic course. Patients who persisted in this treatment for at least one course were analyzed. Result: cured in 214 cases (77.8%), marked by complete disappearance of both symptoms and signs; remarkable effective in 54 cases (19.7%), marked by approximate disappearance of symptoms and signs, or only leaving slight discomfort of the throat; ineffective in 7 cases (2.5%). The total effective rate was 97.5%. The author pointed out that the short-term effect of auricular-point-pressing in treating chronic tonsillitis is satisfactory, while the long-term effect needs further observation.

Remarks

Because chronic tonsillitis has a long duration, intractable symptoms and complex etiology, it is difficult to obtain remarkable improvement or recovery within a short-term treatment. Therefore, 1－2 more courses are needed even when symptoms have disappeared or greatly improved.

During treatment, ask the patient to abstain from pungent food, to give up smoking and drinking and avoid dust and other physico-chemical stimulation.

5. Acute conjunctivitis

Acute conjunctivitis, commonly called *Hong Yan Bing* (Pink-Eye Disease) or *Huo Yan* (Fire Eye), is a contagious eye disease. It occurs mostly in spring and autumn, characterized by obvious congestion of mucopurulent secretion of the eyes. Its main clinical manifestations include photophobia, lacrimation, foreign body and/or burning sensation of the eyes, swelling and pain of the eyelids, congestion of the conjunctiva and profuse eye secretion which is more obvious in the morning after getting up and often sticks the eyelash.

In TCM, acute conjunctivitis belongs to the category of *Tian Xing Chi Yan* (Epidemic Pink Eye). It is believed to be caused by invasion of exogenous Wind-Heat or hyperactive Fire in the Liver and Gallbladder leading to obstruction of Channels and stagnation of Qi and Blood.

Point (Fig. 5—66) and method

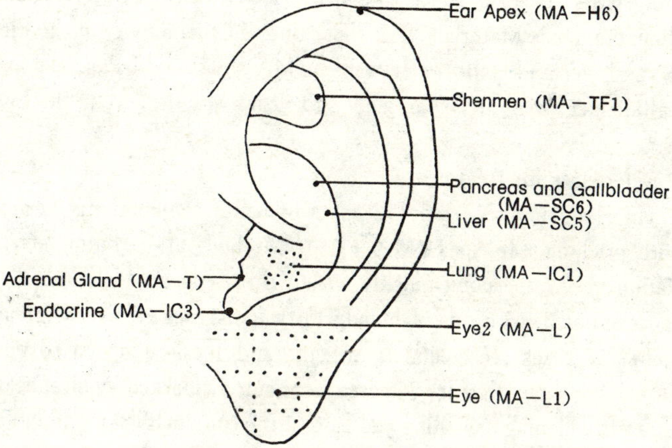

Fig. 5—66 Points for acute conjunctivitis

Main points: Ear Apex (MA—H6), Eye1 (MA—L), Eye2 (MA—L), Shenmen (MA—AT1), Adrenal Gland (MA—T), Endocrine (MA—IC3).

Supplementary points: Lung (MA—IC1), Liver (MA—SC5), Pancreas and Gallbladder (MA—SC6).

Method: Ear Apex (MA—H6) is pricked to cause bleeding. Other points are treated by auricular-point-pressing with vaccaria seeds or cassia seeds. The opposite pressing or perpendicular pressing with strong stimulation is recommended.

Basis for selection of point

This disease should be treated with the therapeutic principle of clearing away Heat, subsiding swelling and relieving pain. Ear Apex (MA—H6), is selected and treated with bloodletting therapy to clear away Heat, to remove Toxic Materials, to subdue swelling and relieve pain. Eye1 (MA—L) and Eye2 (MA—L) are selected as the corresponding points to the diseased part to regulate Qi and Blood in the local area to activate Blood and remove Blood stasis. Shenmen (MA—AT1), Adrenal Gland (MA—T) and Endocrine (MA—IC3) are used to tranquilize the mind and relieve inflammation, swelling and pain. For those due to invasion of exogenous Wind and Heat, Lung (MA—IC1) is added to dispel Wind, to clear away Heat and eliminate Toxic Materials. For those due to hyperactivity of the Fire in the Liver and Gallbladder, Liver (MA—SC5) and Pancreas and Gallbladder (MA—SC6) are added to clear away the Fire in the Liver.

References for treatment

Hu Hongying reported 112 cases of acute conjunctivitis treated with pricking Ear Apex (MA—H6). Method: after routine sterilization, prick the point quickly with a three-edged needle and then squeeze out 3—5 drops of blood. Fifty-four cases received 1 treatment, 58 cases received 2 treatments and 1 case stopped to take herbal medicine. Result: 75 cases were cured, marked by disappearance of reddening, swelling and pain of the conjunctiva, photophobia and profuse eye secretion; 36 cases were improved, marked by obvious improvement of the above symptoms and signs; and 1 failed to respond. The total effective rate was 99.1%.

Jin Zhiying reported 64 cases of hemorrhagic conjunctivitis treated mainly with auricular therapy. Ear Apex (MA—H6) and Eye (MA—L) are selected as main points and Jingming (BL1) as supplemented point. Method: first, puncture Jingming (BL1) with a 1 Cun filiform needle and retain the needle for 15 minutes; then insert a filiform needle into Ear apex (MA—H6) about 0.1 Cun depth and withdraw it 15 minutes later. Squeeze the point immediately to let out several drops of blood. After than, stick a vaccaria seed or green gram on Eye (MA—L1). This treatment was given once daily and the patient was asked to press the stuck seed 10 times every 2—3 hours or so. Result: 44 cases (68.8%) were cured after 1 treatment, 11 cases (17.2%) were cured after 2 treatments and 9 cases (14%) were cured after 3 treatments. The mean recovery time was 48 hours while the time for a spontaneous recovery was 7 times longer—about 2 weeks.

6. Hordeolum

Hordeolum refers to the acute supurative inflammation of the internal or external eyelid due to infection of staphylococcus. It is classified as internal hordeolum and external hordeolum. The external hordeolum occurs in sebaceous glands around ciliary follicles while the internal hordeolum occurs in tarsal glands.

In the beginning, hordeolum is manifested as limited reddening, swelling and pain in the eyelid, which progresses to unmovable localized hard induration like a wheat seed. Several days later, reddening, swelling and pain become worse and a small abscess presents. The abscess will break and then disappear gradually a week later.

In TCM, hordeolum is called *Zhen Yan* (Needle Eye) because it can be cured by being pricked with a needle. TCM holds that this disease is mostly caused by over intake of pungent food leading to retention of Heat in the Spleen and the Stomach, stagnation of Phlegm and Dampness leading to sluggishness of Qi and Blood, or invasion of Wind and Heat into the eyelid.

Point (Fig. 5—67) and method

Main points: Ear Apex (MA—H6), Eye (MA—L1), Liver (MA—SC5), Endocrine (MA—IC3), Adrenal Gland (MA—T).

Supplementary points: Stomach (MA—IC), Spleen (MA—IC), Lung (MA—IC1), Large Intestine (MA—SC4).

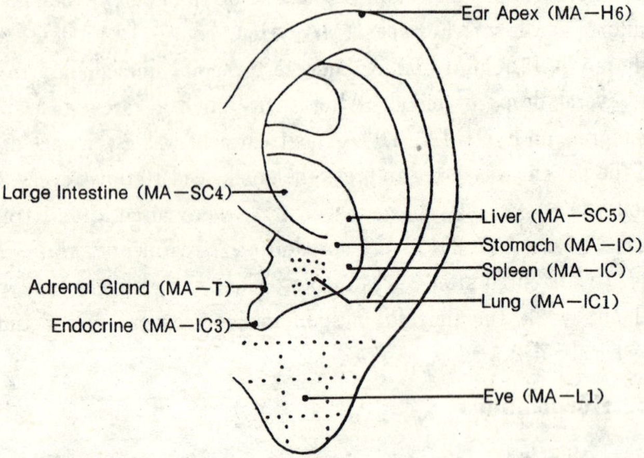

Fig. 5—67 Points for hordeolum

Method: Ear Apex (MA—H6) is pricked to cause bleeding. Other points are treated by auricular-point-pressing with vaccaria seeds. The opposite pressing or perpendicular pressing is recommended.

Basis for selection of point

Ear Apex (MA—H6) is selected and treated with bloodletting therapy to clear away Heat, remove Toxic Materials, subdue swelling and relieve pain. Eye (MA—L1) is selected as the corresponding point to the diseased part. Since the Liver has its specific opening in the eyes, Liver (MA—SC5) is selected to purge the Liver Fire, to activate Blood, to subdue swelling and relieve pain. Endocrine (MA—IC3) and Adrenal Gland (MA—T) have the function of anti-inflammation. The joint use of the above points can reach the aim of clearing away Heat, purging Fire, cooling Blood, removing Toxic Materials, subduing swelling and relieving pain. In case of retention of Heat in the Spleen and the Stomach, Stomach (MA—IC) and Spleen (MA—IC) are added to remove Heat and Dampness, to eliminate Phlegm and resolve masses. In case of invasion of Wind-Heat, Lung (MA—IC1) and Large Intestine (MA—SC4) are added to dispel Wind and clear away Heat.

References for treatment

Yuan Maoxuan reported 50 cases of hordeolum treated with auricular- point-pressing with vaccaria seeds. Points selected were Shenmen (MA—TF1), Kidney (MA—SC), Liver (MA—SC5), Subcortex (MA—AT1), Eye1 (MA—L) and Eye2 (MA—L). The seeds were changed once every other day. During the treatment, ask the patient to press the stuck seeds 2—3 times per day. Result: All of the patients were cured, of which 35 recovered after 1 treatment (2 days), 10 after 2 treatments (4 days), and 5 after 3 treatments (6 days).

Zhao Shengyi reported 50 cases of hordeolum treated with pricking Ear Apex (MA—H6). Method: after routine sterilization, prick the point quickly with a three-edged needle, then squeeze out 3 drops of blood, and then press the point with dry cotton ball. Result: 32 cases were cured, marked by disappearance of symptoms following 2 treatments without administration of any medicine; 14 cases were remarkably improved, marked by recovery following 2 treatments in combination with application of chloromycetin solution; and 4 were ineffectively treated, marked by no response following 2 treatments. The total effective rate was 92%.

7. Myopia

Myopia is a kind of ametropic ophthalmopathy. Without obvious change in the appearance, the diseased eye can see a nearby object clearly but not for those in distance. Clinically, it is classified into two types: true myopia and pseudomyopia. The former results from the condition that the optic axis is too long or the cornea is too powerful in refraction, which causes the external parallel light to be focused before reaching the retina. The latter, also called spasm of the accommodation, is due to overuse of focus adjustment as the result of reading at too close distance. Cyclospasm and the subsequent increase in convexity of lens cause the external parallel light to focalize in front of the retina. These two types can be differentiated through mydriasis despite the same clinical manifestations. After mydriasis, vision will be improved in pseuomyopia but remain unchanged in the true type. Such a disease often bothers young students due to poor illumination, improper sitting posture, overuse or other improper use of eyes.

In TCM, myopia is mostly due to congenital deficiency of the Liver Yin and Kidney Yin and long-term use of eyes impairing Blood, which lead to poor nourishment of the eyes.

Point (Fig. 5—68) and method

Main points: Eye (MA—L1), Eye1 (MA—L), Eye2 (MA—L), Liver (MA—SC5), Kidney (MA—SC).

Supplementary points: Spleen (MA—IC), Subcortex (MA—AT1).

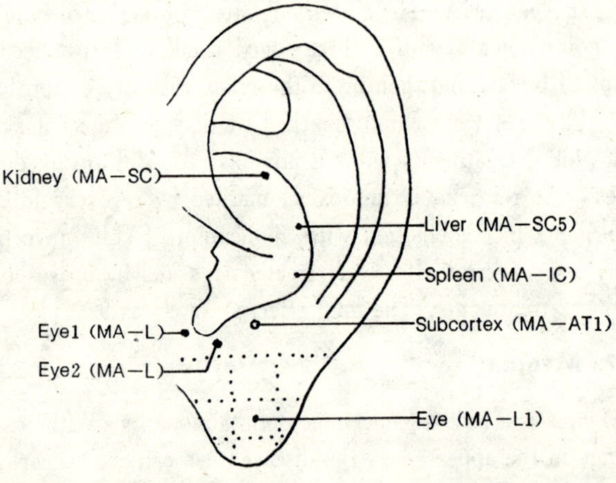

Fig. 5—68 Points for myopia

Method: Mostly apply auricular-point-pressing with vaccaria seeds or magnetic beads. Plaster-sticking therapy can also be applied with those plasters that have strong smell and stimulation such as *She Xiang Zhuang Gu Gao* (Plaster for Strengthening Bone Mainly with Moschus). The perpendicular pressing is recommended.

Basis for selection of point

As corresponding points to the diseased part, Eye (MA—L1), Eye1 (MA—L) and Eye2 (MA—L) are selected to regulate the Channel Qi and improve Blood supply of the eyes. According to TCM theory, the Liver has its specific opening in the eye and stores Blood, the Kidney stores Essence, and the eye functions on the basis of the nourishment of Blood and Essence. Therefore, Liver (MA—SC5) and Kidney (MA—SC) are adopted to reinforce the Liver and the Kidney to enrich Blood and Essence. For pseudomyopia, Spleen (MA—IC) and Subcortex (MA—AT1) are used to ameliorate ciliary adjustment and relieve cyclospasm. In case of strabismus, Gallbladder (MA—SC6) is added.

References for treatment

Jing Renqi observed short-term efficacy of myopia treated with auricular-point-pressing. Total 123 cases (246 eyes) were observed, all of which were students aged between 7—18 years. Points selected were Liver (MA—SC5), Kidney (MA—SC), Eye (MA—L1), Eye1 (MA—L) and Eye2 (MA—L). Vaccaria seeds were used for pressing and the seeds were changed once per week with four treatments constituting one therapeutic course. Vision was re-examined one week after each course. Criteria for effect evaluation: recovery was defined as vision being increased by 4 grades (each line on the visual acuity test chart is stipulated as 1 grade) and having reached 1.0 (equal to 5.0 in international standard); marked improvement was defined as vision being increased by 3 grades but below 1.0; mild improvement was defined as vision being increased by 1—2 grades; and no response was defined as vision increased less than 1 grade. Result: after 1—2 treatment courses, a remarkably effective rate of 30.9% and a total effective rate of 83% were obtained.

Yang Cangliang et al reported 1368 cases (2693 diseased eyes) of myopia treated with auricular-point-pressing. Points selected were Liver (MA—SC5), Eye (MA—L1), Eye1 (MA—L) and Eye2 (MA—L) as main points, Heart (MA—IC), Spleen (MA—IC), Sympathetic (MA—AH7), Shenmen (MA—TF1) and Pancreas and Gallbladder (MA—SC6) as supplementary points. Compound vaccaria seeds used in this treatment were prepared with the following decoction: Semen Vaccariae 1000g, Radix Aconiti Praeparata 30g, Rhizoma Acori Graminei 30g, Borneolum 3g, Camphor 3g. First decoct Radix Aconiti Praeparata 30g, Rhizoma Acori Graminei 30g twice and obtain about 1000 ml of solution, then soak Semen Vaccariae into it, take them out 24 hours later and dry them naturally. Dissolve Borneolum and Camphor in 50 ml of 95% alcoholic solution, and then mix up the solution with the Semen Vaccariae to make compound Semen Vaccariae, which are stored in a sealed container for later use. Treatment was carried out once every other day or every 3 days with alternate use of the two ears. During the treatment, ask the patients to press the stuck seeds several time daily. Eight to ten treatments constituted one therapeutic course and visual acuity was measured at the end of each course. Result: cured in 175 eyes (6. 5%), marked by improvement in visual acuity to 1. 0 above; remarkably effective in 737 eyes (27. 37), marked by visual acuity being increased at least 3 lines in the visual acuity test chart but having not reached 1. 0; mildly effective in 1513 eyes (56. 18%), marked by visual acuity being increased 1—2 lines; and ineffective in 268 eyes (9. 95%). The total effective rate was 90. 05%. A long-term follow-up (2 months to 8 months after treatment was stopped) on 71 cases (141 eyes) revealed that 57 eyes had no reduction in visual acuity (40. 43%), 65 eyes had somewhat reduction in visual acuity but were still better than previous (46. 10%), and 19 eyes had visual acuity reduced to the previous level (13. 55%). The total effective rate was still above 86. 53%. The results indicated that the long-term effect of auricular-point-pressing in treating myopia was also satisfactory.

8. Allergic rhinitis

Allergic rhinitis is an allergic disease of the nasal mucosa caused by allergic reaction due to dust, pollen, food or bacteria. It is mainly manifested as nasal obstruction, watery discharge, sneeze, itching of the nose and hyposmia, accompanied with lacrimation, itching of the eyes, dizziness, headache, itching of the throat and cough.

The characteristic of this disease is sudden onset and withdrawal. During remission period, there is no obvious sign while in attack stage, there are pallor and edema of the nasal mucosa and excess granulocytes in nasal discharge.

In TCM, allergic rhinitis belongs to the category of *Bi Qiu* (Running Nose). It is considered to be caused mostly by invasion of Wind-Cold or other pathogenic factors leading to dysfunction of the Lung Qi and obstruction of the nose. Dysfunction of Zang-Fu organs or deficiency of the Lung, Spleen and Kidney can also contribute to it.

Point (Fig. 5—69) and method

Main points: Internal Nose (MA—T), Lung (MA—IC1), Wind Stream (MA—SF), Adrenal Gland (MA—T), Endocrine (MA—IC3).

Supplementary points: Spleen (MA—IC), Kidney (MA—SC), Forehead (MA—AT), Shenmen (MA—TF1), Pharynx and Larynx (MA—T3).

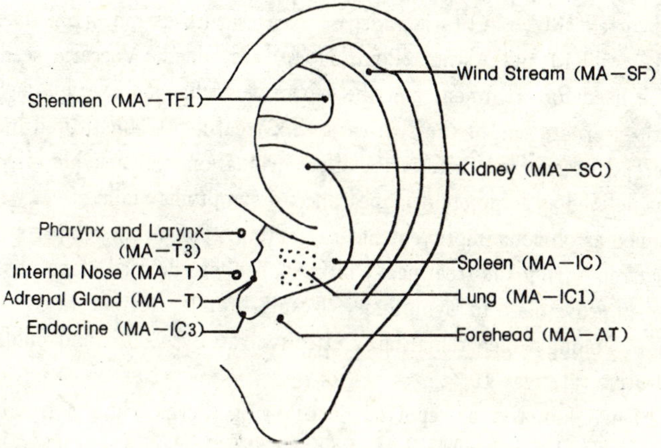

Fig. 5—69 Points for allergic rhinitis

Method: Mostly apply auricular-point-pressing with vaccaria seeds. The opposite pressing or perpendicular pressing is recommended.

Basis for selection of point

As a corresponding point to the diseased part, Internal Nose (MA—T) is selected for removing nasal obstruction. Lung (MA—IC1) and Wind Stream (MA—SF) are selected according to TCM theory to invigorate Qi for strengthening the superficial. Adrenal Gland (MA—AT) and Endocrine (MA—IC3) are selected according to Western medical theory for anti-inflammatory and antiallergic functions. Spleen (MA—IC) and Stomach (MA—IC) and Kidney (MA—SC) are added to tonify the Spleen and the Kidney for invigorating the Lung Qi and strengthening the body resistance against diseases. For those with headache, dizziness and insomnia, Forehead (MA—AT) and Shenmen (MA—TF1) are added. For those with itching in the throat and cough, Pharynx and Larynx (MA—T3) is added.

References for treatment

Qiao Yuling reported 100 cases of allergic rhinitis treated with auricular-point-pressing. Internal Nose (MA—AT), Trachea (MA—IC2) and Lung (MA—IC1) are selected as main points, supplemented with Adrenal Gland (MA—T). For cases with headache, Subcortex (MA—AT1) is added; for cases with asthma, Shenmen (MA—TF1) and Asthma Point (MA) are added. Vaccaria seeds were used for treatment and the seeds were changed every 3 days with alternate use of the two ears. Six treatments constituted one therapeutic course. Criteria for effect evaluation: remarkable effect was defined as complete disappearance of symptoms; mild effect was defined as obvious improvement in symptoms, however, relapse still occurred during the treatment; no response was defined as no obvious improvement in symptoms. Result: total effective rate was 95%, among which remarkably effective rate was 85% and mildly effective rate was 10%.

Shan Qiuhua et al reported 66 cases of allergic rhinitis treated with auricular-point-pressing. Points selected were Lung (MA—IC1), Adrenal Gland (MA—T), Wind Stream (MA—SF), Internal Nose (MA—T), Shenmen (MA—TF1) and Endocrine (MA—IC3). Vaccaria seeds were used for treatment and the seeds were changed every 3—5 days with alternate use of the two ears. Three treatments constituted one therapeutic course. Result: cured in 26 cases, marked by complete disappearance of symptoms after two courses of treatment and no relapse over three months after treatment was discontinued; remarkably effective in 29 cases, marked by complete disappearance of symptoms after two courses of treatment but having relapse within three months after treatment was discontinued; mildly effective in 9 cases, marked by obvious improvement in symptoms after two courses of treatment; and ineffective in 2 cases. The total effective rate was 97%.

9. Tinnitus

Tinnitus, as a common symptom of otopathy, refers to a sound perception in the ear or the head though there is no corresponding sound source in the external environment.

In TCM, the same term is used. It is differentiated as deficiency type and excess type. The former is mostly caused by insufficiency of the Kidney Yin and incoordination between the Kidney and the Heart; while the latter is mostly caused by hyperactivity of the Fire in the Liver and Gallbladder or Phlegm-Fire disturbing the function of the orifice.

Point (Fig. 5—70) and method

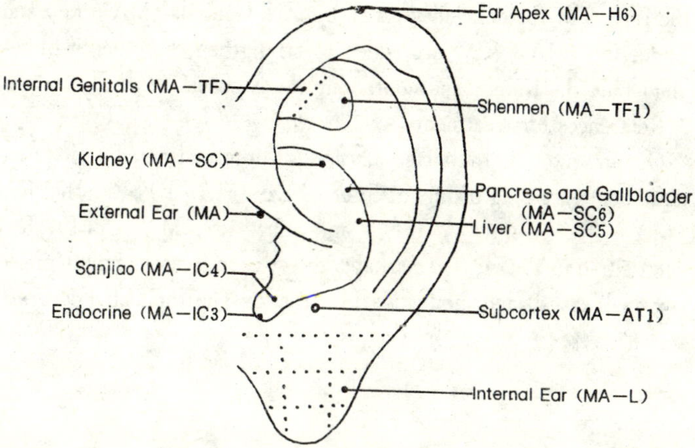

Fig. 5—70 Points for tinnitus

Main points: Internal Ear (MA−L), External Ear (MA−T), Kidney (MA−SC), Sanjiao (MA−IC4), Pancreas and Gallbladder (MA−SC6), Shenmen (MA−TF1), Subcortex (MA−−AT1).

Supplementary points: Liver (MA−SC5), Ear Apex (MA−H6), Internal Genitals (MA−TF), Endocrine (MA−IC3).

Method: Mostly apply auricular-point-pressing with magnetic beads or vaccaria seeds. The perpendicular pressing or intermittent pressing is recommended.

Basis for selection of point

As the corresponding points to the diseased part, Internal Ear (MA−L) and External Ear (MA−T) are selected to improve hearing. The Kidney has its specific opening in the ear, therefore, Kidney (MA−SC) is used to tonify the Kidney and improve hearing. According to the Meridian theory, the Shaoyang Channels enter the ear, so Sanjiao (MA−IC4) and Pancreas and Gallbladder (MA−SC6) are used in combination with Internal Ear (MA−L) and External Ear (MA−T) to regulate Qi and Blood and dredge Channels and Collaterals in the auricular region. Shenmen (MA−TF1) and Subcortex (MA−AT1) are adopted to tranquilize and calm the mind for relieving tinnitus. For the excess type, Liver (MA−SC5) and Ear Apex (MA−H6) are added to clear away the Heat and purge the Fire. For the deficiency type, Internal Genitals (MA−TF) and Endocrine (MA−IC3) are added to strengthen the efficacy of replenishing the Kidney and nourishing the Essence.

References for treatment

Guan Zunxin et al reported 32 cases of tinnitus treated with auricular- point-pressing mainly at Internal Ear (MA−L), External Ear (MA−T), Liver (MA−SC5) and Subcortex (MA−AT1). Result: cured in 12 cases, remarkably effective in 9 cases, mildly effective in 7 cases, and ineffective in 4 cases. The total effective rate was 87.5%.

V. Other Diseases

1. Competitive syndrome

Competitive syndrome refers to a group of symptoms developing before or during competition or examination, such as insomnia, dizziness, palpitation, dysphoria, dry mouth, anorexia, fatigue, lack of concentration, nausea, vomiting, diarrhea or constipation, dysmenorrhea or irregular menstruation, tremor of fingers, cramp of shank and even syncope.

In TCM, this disease is considered to be caused by emotional disturbance, such as fright, fear, anxiety and worry, leading to incoordination between Qi and Blood and dysfunction of Zang-Fu organs and Channels.

Point (Fig. 5—71) and method

Main points: Subcortex (MA—AT1), Shenmen (MA—TF1), Heart (MA—IC), Kidney (MA—SC).

Supplementary points: Occiput (MA—AT), Anterior Ear Lobe (MA—L), Stomach (MA—IC), Spleen (MA—IC), Liver (MA—SC5), Endocrine (MA—IC3).

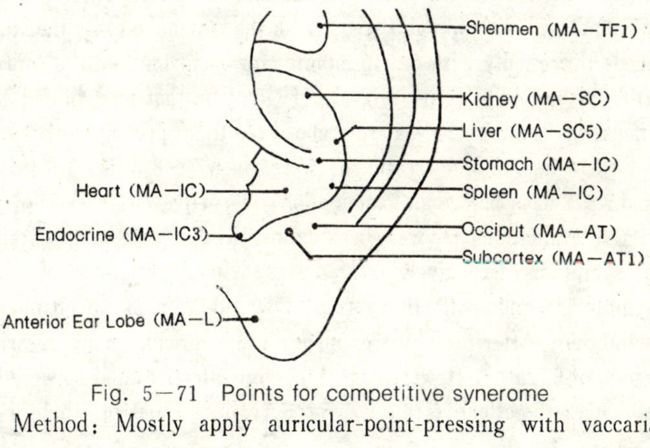

Fig. 5—71 Points for competitive synerome

Method: Mostly apply auricular-point-pressing with vaccaria

seeds, magnetic beads, *Bing Pian* (borneol) or some other seeds. The perpendicular pressing is recommended.

Basis for selection of point

Subcortex (MA—AT1) and Shenmen (MA—TF1) are selected to regulate the excito-inhibitory function of the cerebral cortex and tranquilize the mind. Since the Heart dominates mental activities, Heart (MA—IC) is used to reinforce the Heart and tranquilize the mind. Since the Kidney stores Essence and produces Marrow, Kidney (MA—SC) is used to replenish the Kidney and brain. The joint use of the above points can strengthen the cerebral function and improve psychic stage. For those with insomnia and dizziness, Occiput (MA—AT) and Anterior Ear Lobe (MA—L) are added; for those with anorexia, vomiting and nausea, Stomach (MA—IC) and Spleen (MA—IC) are added; for those with tremor of fingers and cramp of shank, Liver (MA—SC5) and Spleen (MA—IC) are added; and for those with dysmenorrhea and irregular menstruation, Endocrine (MA—IC3) is added.

References for treatment

Zhou Rongyi reported 105 cases of competitive syndrome treated with auricular-point-pressing. All of the subjects were allocated randomly into two groups: the auricular-point-pressing group and the control group. In the auricular-point-pressing group, Heart (MA—IC), Shenmen (MA—TF1) and Subcortex (MA—AT1) were pressed with vaccaria seeds. Ask the patient to press the stuck seeds thrice daily with 5—10 minutes for each time. In the control group, the non-effective mixture of Gentiana that was diluted 100 times was administered as a placebo three times per day with 10 ml for each time. Three treatments were given 7—8 days, 3—4 days and 1—2 days before an examination, respectively. Criteria for effective evaluation: recovery was defined as complete disappearance of symptoms; effectively treated was defined as improvement of symptoms; and ineffectively treated was defined as no change of symptoms. After the first treatment, in the auricular-point-pressing group of 67 cases, 10 were cured, 42 were effective, and 15 were ineffective; the effective rate was 77.6%. In the control group of 50 cases, the effective rate was 68.4%. The total effective rate was 74.3%. After the second treatment, in the auricular-point-pressing group of 37 cases, 21 were cured, 15 were effectively treated, and 1 was ineffectively treated; the effective rate was 97.4%. In the control group of 16 cases, the effective rate was 81.3%. The total effective rate was 92.5%. By comparison, there was a remarkably significant difference ($P<0.01$) in favor of the second treatment. Comparing the effective rates of the two therapies, there was no significant difference after the first treatment, however, there was a significant difference ($P<0.05$) after the second treatment.

Que Yuntai reported 111 cases of competitive syndrome treated with auricular-point-pressing. Main points selected were Heart (MA – IC), Shenmen (MA – TF1), Subcortex (MA – AT1), Spleen (MA–IC) and Occiput (MA–AT). Point -Pressing treatment with Fructus Viticis Neggundo was given 6 days prior to an examination and the stuck seeds were kept until the end of the examination. During this period, ask the patient to press the seeds 3–5 times daily with 10–20 minutes for each time. Result: remarkably effective in 70 cases (63.1%), marked by disappearance of symptoms and 6–8 hours' sleep each night 3 days after the treatment; mildly effective in 33 cases (29.17%), marked by obvious improvement of symptoms and over 5 hours' sleep each night; and ineffective in 8 cases (7.2%). The total effective rate was 92.8%.

Remarks

To prevent competitive syndrome, it is suggested that auricular-point- pressing therapy be given 3–5 days before competition.

2. Transfusion reaction

Transfusion reaction is an allergic reaction caused by exogenous or endogenous pyrogen, mostly occurring when fluid or blood has been infused 100–200 ml. It is manifested as a sudden onset of chill, aching pain of joints, pallor of skin, cyanosis, and subsequent high fever. The fever may reach 39℃ or higher and last 2–3 hours, then it abates following perspiration and leaves fatigue, muscular soreness and heaviness behind. A few patients may present itching, urticaria, angioneurotic edema, and even chest distress, asthma and spasm and edema of the larynx. Mild transfusion reaction brings about sufferings to the patient while a severe one may endanger the patient's life. Therefore, it is of great significance to prevent transfusion reaction.

Point (Fig. 5−72) and method

Points: Adrenal Gland (MA−T), Wind Stream (MA−SF), Endocrine (MA−IC3), Shenmen (MA−TF1), Apex of Antitragus (MA−AT).

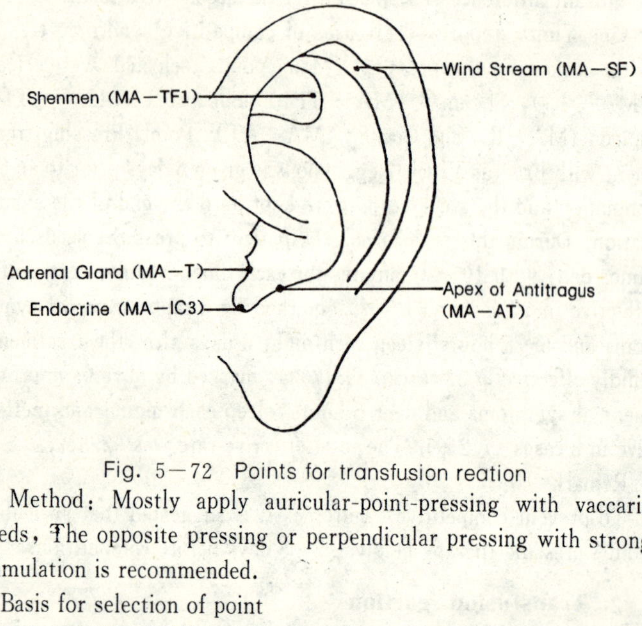

Fig. 5−72 Points for transfusion reation

Method: Mostly apply auricular-point-pressing with vaccaria seeds, The opposite pressing or perpendicular pressing with strong stimulation is recommended.

Basis for selection of point

Adrenal Gland (MA−T), Wind Stream (MA−SF) and Endocrine (MA−IC3) are three important antiallergic points. Therefore, they are used jointly to strengthen the antiallergic function, to inhibit capillary exudation, antigen-antibody reaction in the skin, mucosa and Blood and release of histamine, and to relieve spasm of smooth muscle. Shenmen (MA−TF1) and Apex of Antitragus (MA−AT) are used to tranquilize and calm the mind.

References for treatment

Zhang Guiming reported 99 cases of transfusion reaction treated with auricular needling at Shenmen (MA－TF1), Adrenal Gland (MA－T) and Heart (MA－IC). Filiform needles were used to puncture the selected points. Result: excellently effective in 79 cases, marked by withdrawal of reaction 3 minutes after insertion of needles; remarkably effective in 17 cases, marked by withdrawal of reaction 3—5 minutes after insertion of needles; mildly effective in 3 cases, marked by withdrawal of reaction 5—17 minutes after insertion of needles.

Remarks

Auricular-point-pressing proves quite effective for preventing transfusion reaction. The treatment can be given 5—10 minutes prior to transfusion.

In case of severe reaction, it is necessary to apply other kinds of therapy simultaneously.

3. Motion sickness

Motion sickness is manifested as nausea, vomiting, pale complexion and cold sweating during traveling by car, ship or plane. Western medicine believes that it results from influence of some kinds of movement on the semicircular canals.

In TCM, motion sickness belongs to the categories of Xuan Yun (Dizziness) and Ou Tu (Vomiting). It is considered to be associated with deficiency of the Spleen and the Stomach or high sensitivity to special smell such as that of gasoline.

Point (Fig. 5—73) and method

Main points: Occiput (MA—AT), Shenmen (MA—TF1), Cardia (MA—IC7), Stomach (MA—IC), Subcortex (MA—AT1).

Supplementary points: Wind Stream (MA—SF), Endocrine (MA—IC3).

Method: Mostly apply auricular-point-pressing with vaccaria seeds, *She Xiang Zhuang Gu Gao* (Plaster for Strengthening Bone Mainly with Moschus) can be used for sticking seeds. The opposite pressing or perpendicular pressing is recommended.

Basis for selection of point

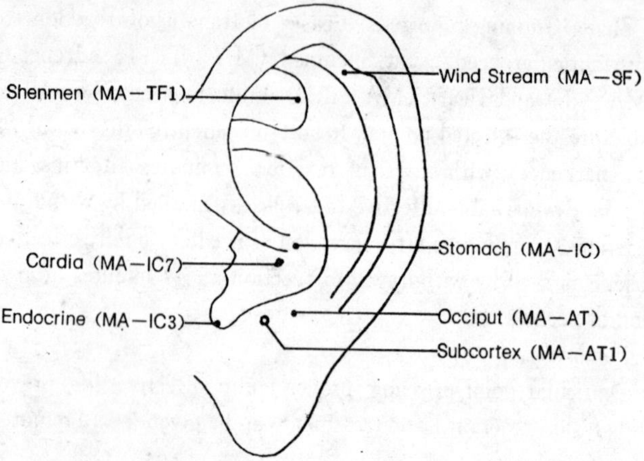

Fig. 5—73 Points for motion sickness

Occiput (MA—AT) is a key point for relieving dizziness. Shenmen (MA — TF1) is used to tranquilize and calm the mind and strengthen the efficacy of relieving dizziness. Cardia (MA—IC7) and Stomach (MA—IC) are selected to send down the adverse flow of the Stomach Qi to stop vomiting. Subcortex (MA—AT1) is used to regulate the cerebral cortical function, to tranquilize the mind and arrest vomiting as well. For cases resulting from stimulation of gasoline, Wind Stream (MA—SF) and Endocrine (MA—IC3) are added to strengthen antiallergic function.

References for treatment

Wang Zhaojie et al reported 91 cases of motion sickness treated with auricular-point-pressing. Of them, 51 cases recovered, 35 cases improved, and 5 cases did not respond. The total effective rate was 94.5%. Comparative study showed that auricular therapy is superior to theohydraminum and topical application.

4. Withdrawal from smoking

Auricular-point-pressing can eliminate the smoker's addiction to cigarette and relieve withdrawal symptoms such as lassitude, restlessness, discomfort sensation of the throat, frequent yawning, palpitation, headache and vomiting.

Point (Fig. 5—74) and method

Main points: Lung (MA—IC1), Mouth (MA—IC5), Shenmen (MA—TF1), Subcortex (MA—AT1).

Supplementary points: Heart (MA—IC), Liver (MA—SC5), Stomach (MA—IC), Occiput (MA—AT), Pharynx and Larynx (MA—T3).

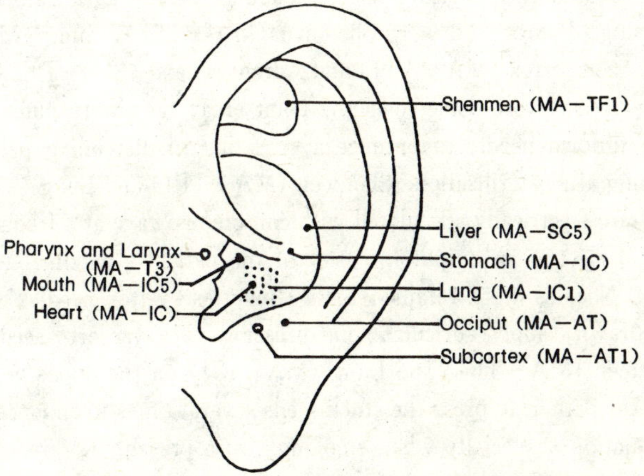

Fig. 5—74 Points for withdrawal from smoking

Method: Mostly apply auricular-point-pressing with vaccaria seeds, The opposite pressing or perpendicular pressing is recommended.

Basis for selection of point

The desire for smoking results from conditional reflex which develops from long-term stimulation on nicotine to the afferent nerve of the receptor of the respiratory tract, subsequently leading to development of excitatory center in the cerebral cortex. Therefore, Lung (MA—IC1) and Mouth (MA—IC5) are selected to inhibit the reflex and regulate the Lung Qi. Shenmen (MA—TF1) and Subcortex (MA—AT1) function to tranquilize the mind and regulate the cerebral cortical function to check the smoking excitatory center and block the conditional reflex, thus reaching the purpose of giving up smoking. For those complaining of palpitation and restlessness, Heart (MA—IC) and Liver (MA—SC5) are added; for those complaining of headache and nausea, Stomach (MA—IC) and Occiput (MA—AT) are added; and for those complaining of discomfort sensation of the throat, Pharynx and Larynx (MA—T3) is added.

References for treatment

Chen Xiuzhen et al reported 63 cases of quitting smoking. They were treated with auricular electroacupuncture and auricular-point-pressing. Points used were Shenmen (MA—TF1), Lung (MA—IC1), Subcortex (MA—AT1) and Adrenal Gland (MA—T). After tender spots were detected in the point area, they were punctured with filiform needle to produce a sensation of distending pain or burning after sterilization. Shenmen (MA—TF1) and Lung (MA—IC1) are electrically stimulated with continuous wave at a frequency of 200 Hz and an output intensity of the patient's maximal tolerance. Needles were retained for 30 minutes. After needles were withdrawn, apply auricular-point-pressing with vaccaria seeds at Shenmen (MA—TF1) and Lung (MA—IC1) on the opposite ear. Ask the patient to press the stuck seeds several times to enhance the stimulation, especially when smoking desire presented. Treatment was performed once daily with 7 treatments constituting one therapeutic course. Result: remarkably effective in 25 cases (39.68%), marked by withdrawal of smoking; mildly effective in 22 cases (34.92%), marked by smoking being reduced to 4—7 cigarettes per day; and ineffective in 9 cases (14.29%).

Li Huanbin reported 63 cases of quitting smoking. They were treated with auricular-point-pressing. Result: successful withdrawal of smoking in 11 cases, remarkably effective in 9 cases, mildly effective in 6 cases, and ineffective in 2 cases. Measurement of sulfocyanate (SCN) in saliva revealed that the content of SCN was reduced from a mean value of 75 ng/ml to zero after the smokers gave up smoking with the help of this treatment. There was a significant difference before and after treatment. The mean content of SCN was zero in both non-smokers and those who had given up smoking, and there was no significant difference between them.

耳穴贴压疗法
单秋华 著
陆明霞
肖 飞 译
*
山东科学技术出版社出版
中国济南市玉函路 16 号 邮政编码 250002
中国山东莱芜市印刷厂印刷
中国国际图书贸易总公司发行
中国北京车公庄西路 35 号
北京邮政信箱第 399 号 邮政编码 100044
*
1996 年(大 32 开) 1 版 1 次
ISBN 7－5331－1833－2
R·529
07200
14－E－3024P